The Mixed Martial Arts Handbook

The Mixed Martial Arts Handbook

The Insider's Guide to Fighting Techniques

John Ritschel

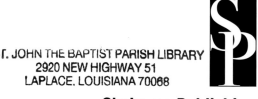

Skyhorse Publishing

Skyhorse Publishing books may be purchased in bulk at special discounts for sales promotion, corporate gifts, fund-raising, or educational purposes. Special editions can also be created to specifications. For details, contact the Special Sales Department, Skyhorse Publishing, 555 Eighth Avenue, Suite 903, New York, NY 10018 or info@skyhorsepublishing.com.

www.skyhorsepublishing.com

10 9 8 7 6 5 4 3 2 1

Library of Congress Cataloging-in-Publication Data

Ritschel, John.
  The mixed martial arts handbook : the insider's guide to fighting techniques / John Ritschel.
      p. cm.
  Includes index.
  ISBN 978-1-60239-792-7
  1. Mixed martial arts. I. Title.
  GV1102.7.M59R47 2009
  796.815--dc22
                          2009039119

Disclaimer: It is always the responsibility of the individual to assess his or her own fitness capability before participating in any training activity. While every effort has been made to ensure the content of this is as technically accurate as possible, neither the author nor the publishers can accept responsibility for any injury or loss sustained as a result of the use of this material.

Printed in China

Contents

ACKNOWLEDGMENTS

I would like to thank my partner Jane for supporting me in writing this book. She played an integral part in making sure the explanations in the book were not too technical and would be understood by someone new to mixed martial arts. I would also like to thank her for her support and understanding while I was competing. Her words were always my strongest weapon.

My thanks also go out to the guys at the Olympik Dream gym for giving us their full support during the photo shoot.

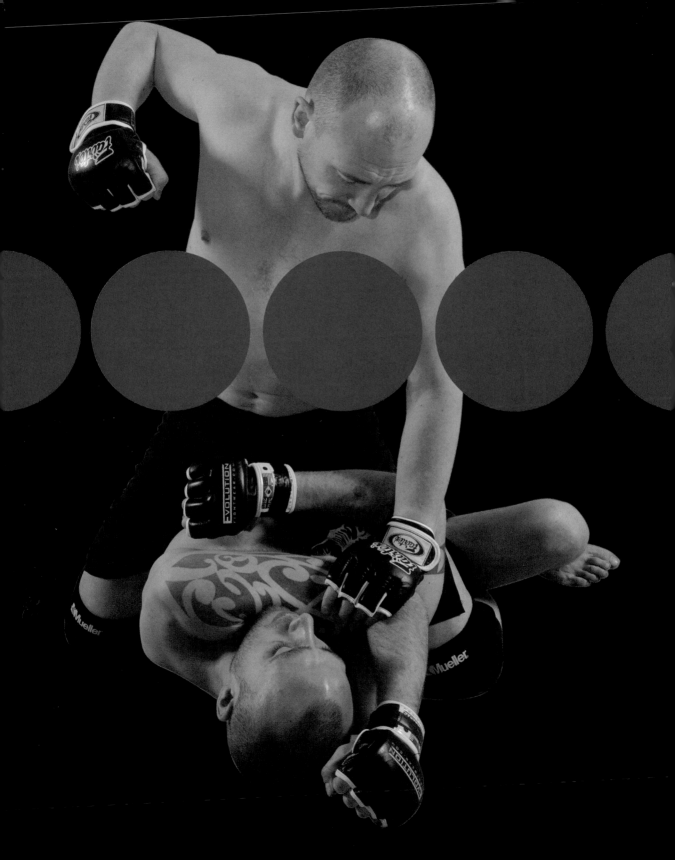

INTRODUCTION

Mixed Martial Arts (MMA) is a full-contact martial art and allows a wide variety of techniques, from striking to grappling. What makes MMA unique is that striking is allowed when standing and when on the ground. In other combat martial arts, such as kick-boxing and Thai boxing, if a competitor goes to the ground the fight stops until both fighters are back on their feet.

MMA became popular when the Ultimate Fighting Championship (UFC) was founded in 1993. The competition's aim was to find the most effective martial arts by letting competitors from different fighting backgrounds compete with minimal rules; it was also known as 'no-holds-barred'. However current UFC rules have been adapted to safeguard competitors.

The previous martial arts background of a MMA fighter will dictate their preferred techniques as well as their strengths and weaknesses.

Strikers rely on punches, kicks, elbows and knees to knock out their opponent and they tend to have a background in Thai boxing, kick-boxing, boxing or karate.

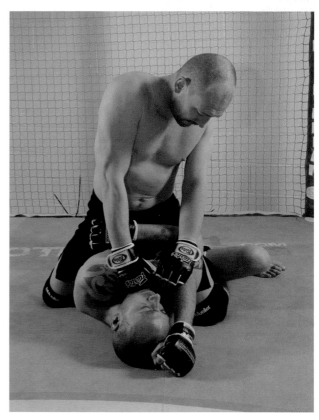

Fig 0.1 A fighter striking an opponent while they are on the ground.

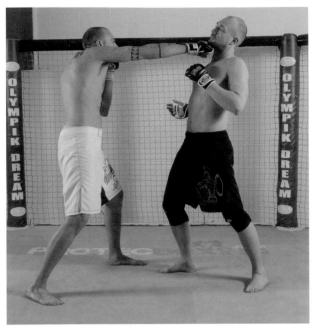

Fig 0.2A A right cross.

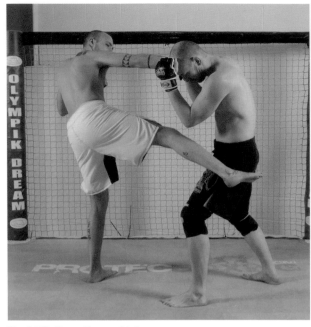

Fig 0.2B Roundhouse kick.

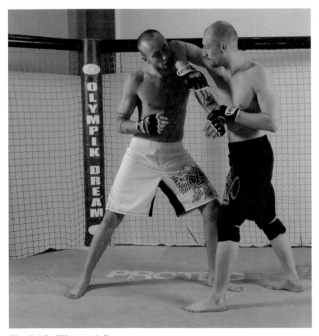

Fig 0.2C Elbow strike.

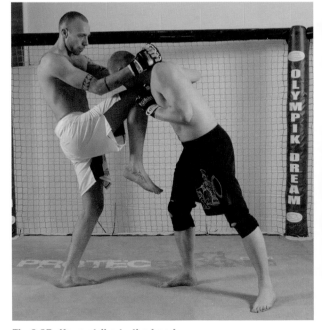

Fig 0.2D Knee strike to the head.

Wrestlers rely on takedowns and 'Ground and pound' (see Chapter 4). Their previous experience would be in one of the different styles of wrestling, for example Greco-Roman or freestyle. The main techniques used would be clinching, holding, locking, and leverage.

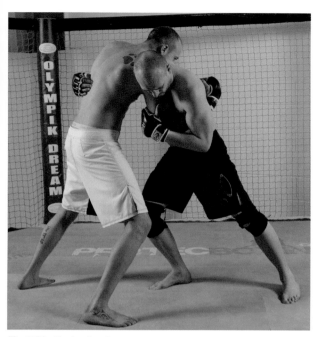

Fig 0.3A Under hook.

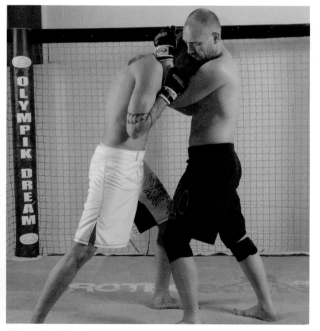

Fig 0.3B Thai clinch.

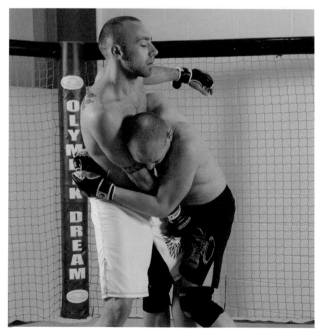

Fig 0.3C A hold.

Submission competitors rely on gaining a hold or lock to force the opponent to 'tap out', thus preventing injury or pain. The submission is commonly performed by clearly tapping the floor or the opponent. Previous disciplines for these could include Brazilian jiu-jitsu, judo or sambo. The main techniques fighters used would be choke holds, compression locks and joint locks.

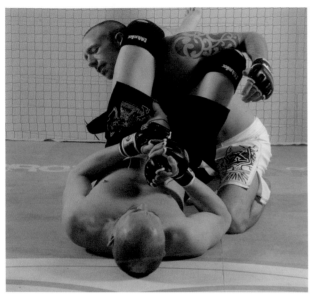

Fig 0.4A Arm bar.

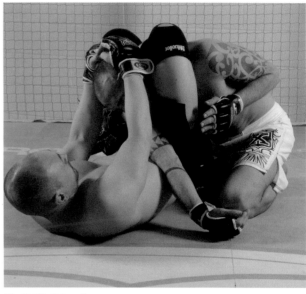

Fig 0.4B Triangle.

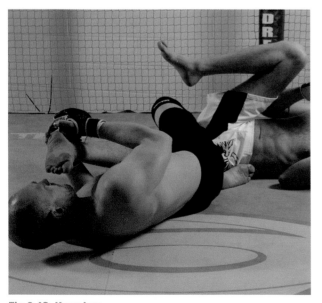

Fig 0.4C Knee bar.

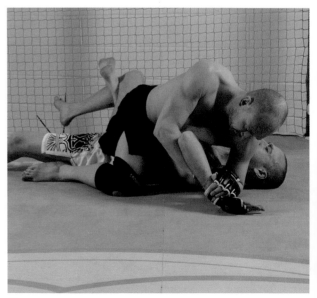

Fig 0.4D Americana.

Whatever background a fighter is from, it is important that they learn and incorporate moves from other styles too, as MMA is based on exploitation of weaknesses and the application of strengths. Fighting strategies are specific to an opponent and an effective fighter is one that can adapt in this way while minimising their own weaknesses and maximising their own strengths.

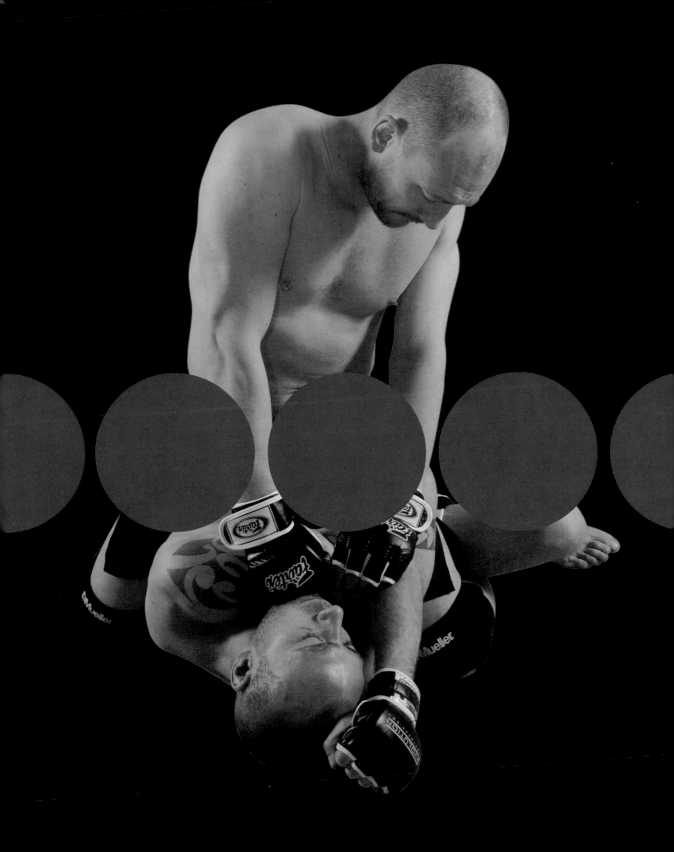

CHAPTER **ONE**
The history of mixed martial arts

A sport similar to modern MMA can be found in Greek mythology. Known as *pankration*, it is said to have been invented by the Greek heroes Heracles and Theseus. Pankration combined wrestling and boxing and was included in the Olympic Games in 648 BC. Legend has it that pankration was also part of the training for the famous Spartans.

A more recent example is the martial art known as *bartitsu*, which was founded in London in 1899 and combined Asian and European fighting styles.

However, modern MMA traces its roots back to Brazil and the Gracie family's *Vale Tudo* tournaments, which started in the 1920s. The 'Gracie Challenge' became famous for its limited rules; Vale Tudo, when translated, literally means 'anything goes'.

There was also the 'shoot-style' movement in Japanese professional wrestling, which led to the formation of the first MMA organisation in 1985. Interest continued to grow in Japan and the first PRIDE Fighting Championship took place in 1997 with a similar ethos to Vale Tudo.

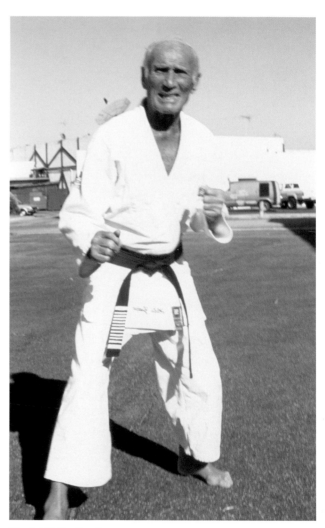

Fig 1.1 Helio Gracie.

In 1993 the sport's popularity increased again following Royce Gracie's win in the first-ever Ultimate Fighting Championship (UFC) held in the United States. UFC was born from the concept of matching fighters from different styles with minimal rules to determine the most effective in a real-life combat situation. However, current MMA rules have been adapted to minimise potential injury.

Today the UFC is recognised globally as the largest promoter of MMA and is shown on TV in over 30 countries worldwide.

MMA, as one of the fastest-growing combat sports in the world, has also been debated for future inclusion in the Olympic Games. The International Olympic Committee has notified the world governing bodies of seven sports that they will be considered for inclusion at the 2016 Summer Olympics. The sports are baseball, softball, golf, rugby, karate, roller sports and squash, but there is only room for two new sports, so competition is fierce. In October 2009, the IOC will decide the final schedule for 2016 during its Copenhagen session.

The pressure on the International Olympic Committee to include MMA is gaining momentum, not least from the athletes themselves. The Japanese Judo Olympic gold

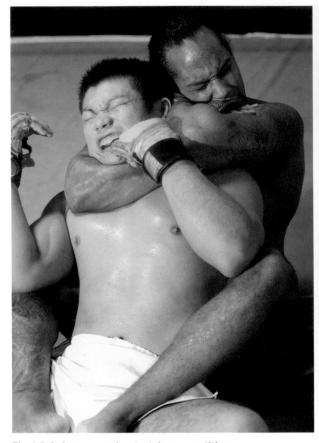

Fig 1.2 A Japanese shoot-style competition.

medallist of the 2008 Beijing Games, Satoshi Ishii has announced a move into the cash-rich world of mixed martial arts and Ben Askren, a 2008 Olympic wrestler has also stated that he will either compete again as a wrestler in the 2012 Olympics, or make his move into the world of MMA. Such high profile names entering the sport will surely add weight to the argument for Olympic inclusion in the future.

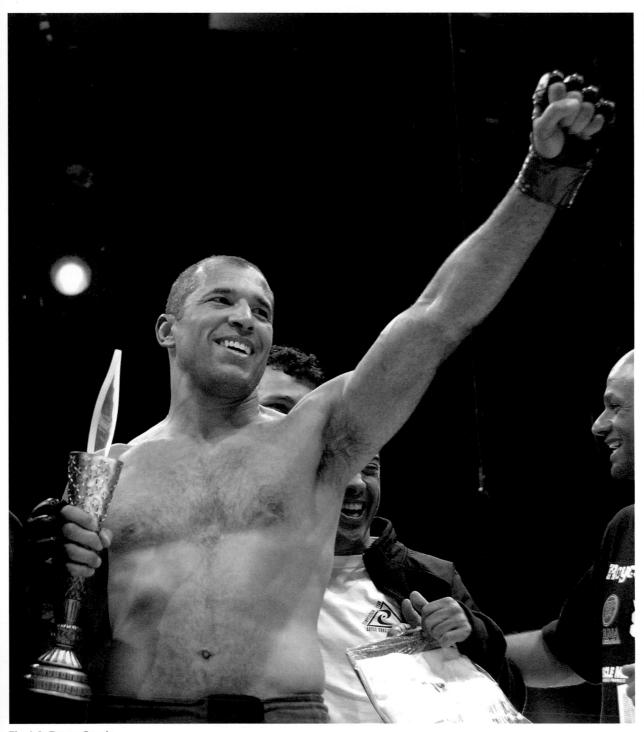

Fig 1.3 Royce Gracie.

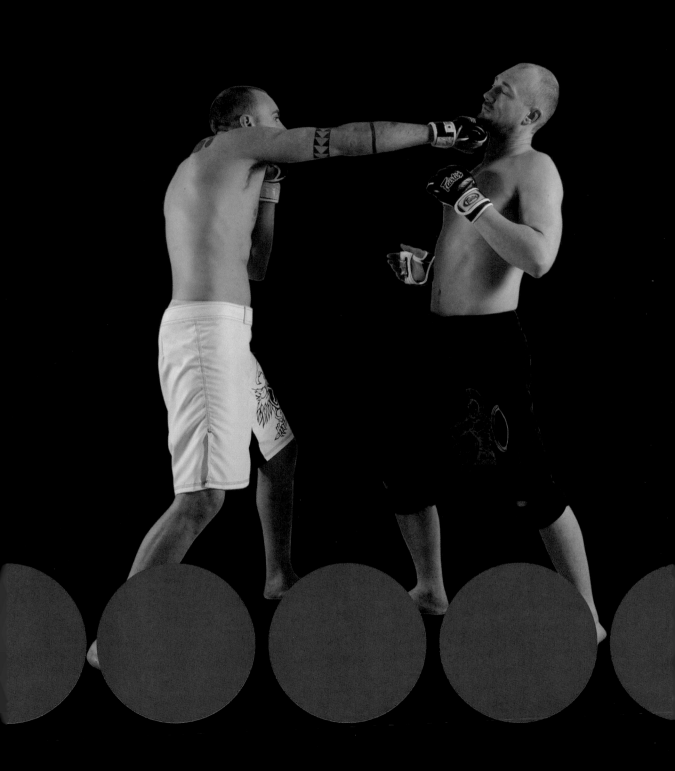

CHAPTER **TWO**
Mixed martial arts in competition

MMA is usually split into three different categories – amateur, semi-professional and professional – and then by weight.

Amateurs can wear shin protection and gloves that are slightly more padded, and are not allowed to strike an opponent who is on the ground. However, bouts are still full contact and, depending on the organisers, head strikes may or may not be allowed when standing.

Below you can see the difference between normal boxing gloves (Fig 2.1) and MMA gloves (Fig 2.2). The boxing gloves have more padding, while the MMA gloves normally have the thumb and fingertips exposed as this increases the number of techniques that can be used, for example a choke hold.

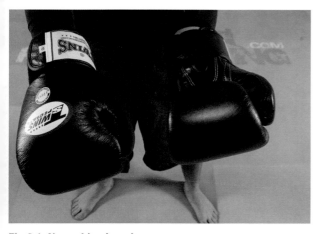

Fig 2.1 Normal boxing gloves.

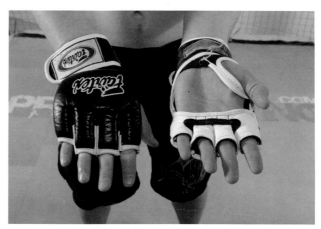

Fig 2.2 MMA gloves.

Semi-professional bouts have all the elements of a professional match, however the rules can be negotiated between the different instructors. Weight classes can also vary hugely between different organisations. The professionals have full MMA rules, including gloves with less padding and no shin protection.

The professional and semi-professional fights take place in an eight-sided cage (*see* Fig 2.3), while the amateur bouts are fought on a mat. To win, one of the competitors has to knock out their opponent or have them resign by tapping out.

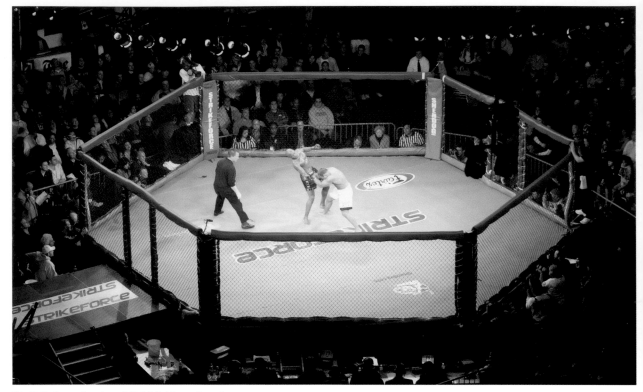

Fig 2.3 A professional fight taking place in a cage.

Competition rules

The rules of MMA competitions have changed over the years both to move the sport away from its previous barbaric image of no-holds-barred, and to protect the fighters. Changes have ranged from the introduction of weight classes to the use of small open-fingered gloves to protect the fists and minimise stoppages due to cuts. Time limits have also been introduced to curtail fights with little action in which fighters were conserving their energy. If a referee feels that both competitors are resting rather than fighting on the ground, they can make them stand and restart the fight.

Again, rules can be specific to associations, but there is usually a common theme to allow fighters to easily adapt.

Victory

A bout can be won in one of five ways:

Knockout (KO) If a fighter becomes unconscious due to a heavy blow, the fight is stopped and the fighter who delivered the blow is declared the winner.

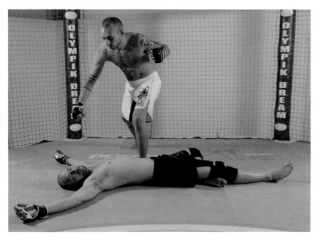

Fig 2.4 Knockout.

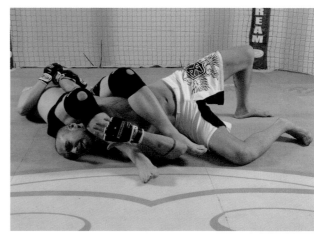

Fig 2.5 Submission – 'tapping out'.

Submission A fighter can admit defeat by 'tapping out'. The tap can be against the opponent's body, the mat or the floor. The fighter can also verbally declare defeat.

Technical knockout (TKO) A referee may stop a fight if one competitor becomes dominant to the point that their opponent cannot protect themselves, if they become unconscious from a hold or if they develop significant injuries. The referee can call a doctor for an assessment of injuries and, if declared severe, the fight can be stopped.

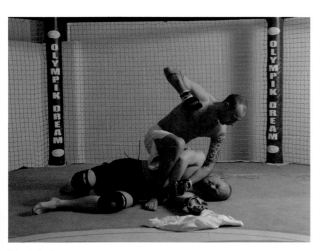

Fig 2.6 Corner stoppage.

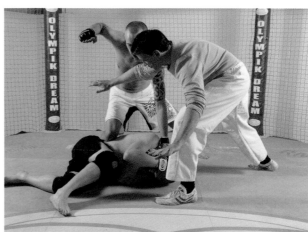

Fig 2.7 Stoppage by the referee.

Corner stoppage Each fighter has their own coach standing in their corner during a bout. The coach can stop the fight at any time by literally throwing in the towel. A coach will often do this to protect their fighter.

Referee's decision If all the bouts are completed, a panel of three judges decides the winner. A referee can also disqualify a fighter if they commit three fouls during a fight.

Fouls

The following actions are commonly viewed as fouls:

- hair pulling;
- biting;
- eye gouging;
- headbutting;
- fish-hooking (where the fighter hooks their finger into their opponent's mouth and pulls);
- choking an opponent for longer than three seconds;
- small joint manipulation (where toes and fingers are twisted or bent, giving a weaker opponent the advantage);
- strikes to the back of the head, groin and spinal or kidney areas.

Rounds

The number and duration of rounds varies depending on the association and type of competition. Most consist of three rounds of five minutes each with a minute's break in between. However, title fights can last for five rounds.

Safety equipment and uniform

All fighters must wear the following safety equipment:

- groin guard;
- gum shield;
- 4–6 ounce gloves that allow the fingers to grab.

The common uniform consists of approved shorts. Cotton gis such as karate/judo-style suits are not normally allowed.

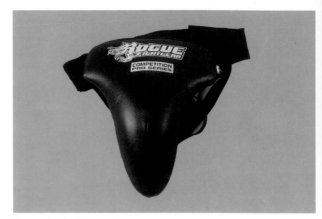

Fig 2.8A Groin guard.

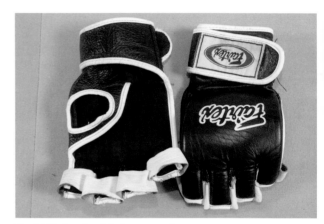

Fig 2.8B A pair of 4–6 ounce gloves.

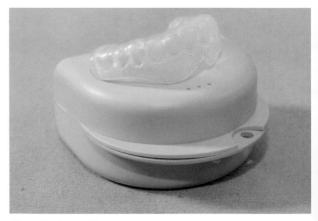

Fig 2.8C Gum shield.

Grading

Unlike the more traditional martial arts, MMA doesn't have a standard grading system used by each of the different governing bodies and associations.

Categories

In most amateur and professional competitions fighters are matched by weight. Although these categories can vary between associations, the most common are shown here.

The UFC is setting the benchmark in martial arts and currently uses the five weight classes from Lightweight to Heavyweight. Other associations vary – DREAM is a Japanese Mixed Martial Arts promoter with 6 weight categories, each with a champion with a defendable title. The bouts used by this promoter also differ, with 10 minutes for the first round and 5 minutes for the second round.

WEIGHT CLASS NAME	UPPER LIMIT lb	EQUIVALENT kg
Flyweight	125	57
Bantamweight	135	61
Featherweight	145	66
Lightweight	155	70
Welterweight	170	77
Middleweight	185	84
Light heavyweight	205	93
Heavyweight	265	120
Super heavyweight	No upper weight limit	

Table 2.1 The most common MMA weight categories.

Optimal competition weight

A fighter's optimal competing weight is less than their normal everyday weight, with emphasis placed on being stronger, faster and fitter than the opponent. However, it is important that this is achieved without exhaustion setting in and therefore a healthy eating plan should be followed.

Preparations ideally start eight weeks prior to competing, with the last two or three kilograms being lost in a sauna the day before the weigh-in. Reducing weight by restricting food and water intake is not an effective method as this also reduces stamina and performance levels.

A fighter should always be well rested and properly fuelled and hydrated before a competition.

Conditioning for competitions

Endurance and short-burst cardiovascular interval training are both important preparations for competition. Endurance can be achieved by running long distances, and sprinting is a good form of high-intensity interval training.

However, the very best preparation is to spar with training partners as this teaches technical finesse as well as building mental and physical stamina. This method also trains the fighter to remain effective when they become fatigued in a real competition.

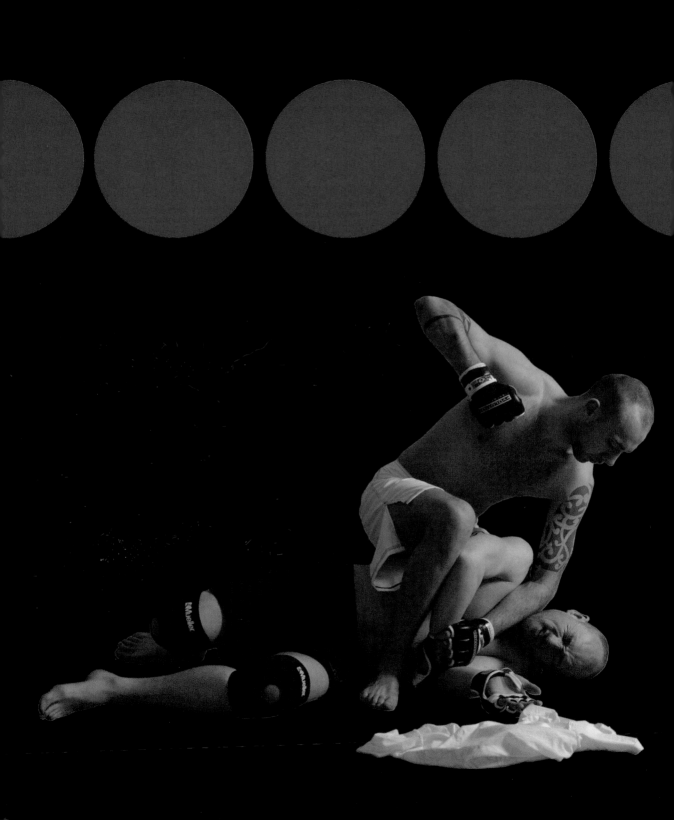

CHAPTER **THREE**
Adaptation of traditional martial arts techniques

MMA bouts start with both competitors standing and therefore benefits fighters who use striking techniques such as punching, kicking, elbowing and kneeing.

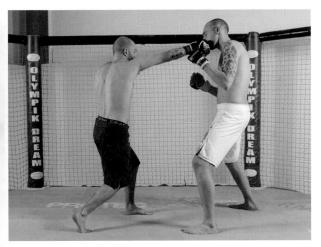

Fig 3.1 Boxing and punching techniques.

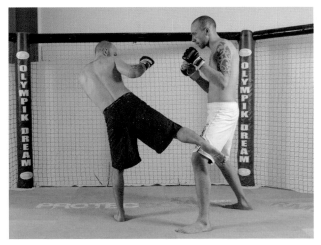

Fig 3.2 Roundhouse kicking techniques to the knee.

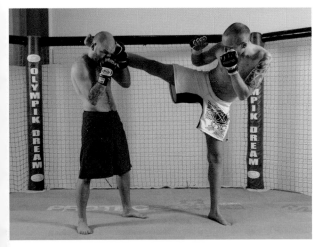

Fig 3.3 Kicking techniques to the body and head.

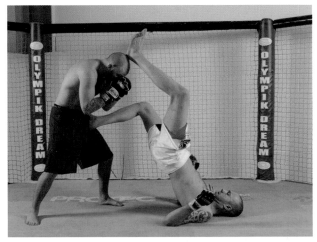

Fig 3.4 Kicking techniques from the ground.

MMA is one of the few martial arts to allow kicks both to the upper knee and to an opponent while they are on the floor. Examples of both can be seen below, along with elbowing and kneeing techniques.

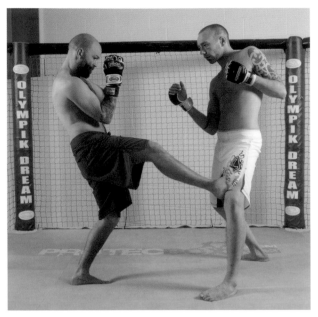

Fig 3.5 Stomp to the knee.

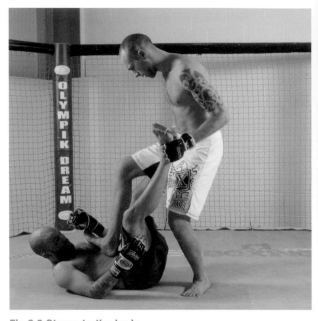

Fig 3.6 Stomp to the body.

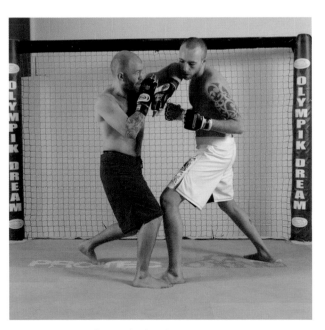

Fig 3.7 Elbow strike to the head.

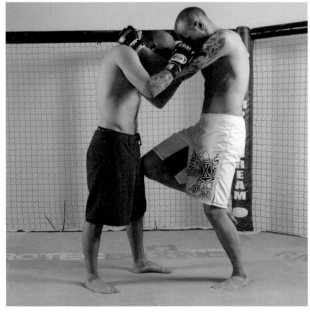

Fig 3.8 Knee strike to the upper thigh.

However, standing fighting can quickly become stand-up grappling or clinching. Striking techniques can also be applied from these positions.

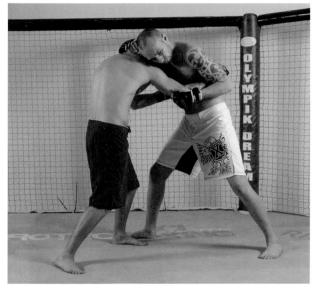

Fig 3.9 Stand-up grappling.

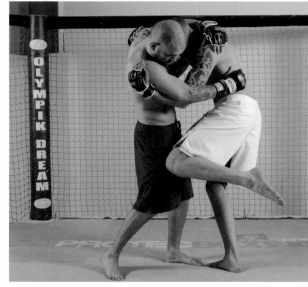

Fig 3.10 Clinching technique.

When the fight is taken to the ground, a variety of ground grappling techniques can be utilised such as choke holds, arm bars, leg bars or pinning techniques. These methods can also be combined with striking techniques.

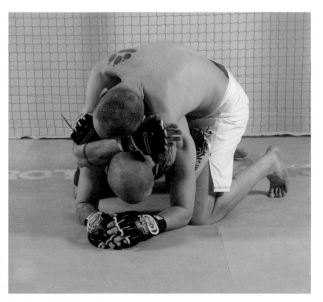

Fig 3.11 Choke hold.

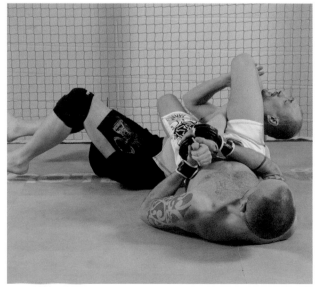

Fig 3.12 Arm bar.

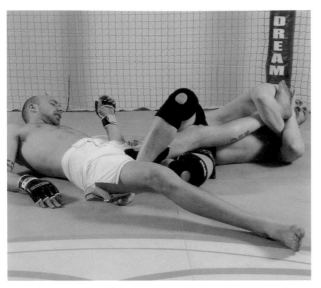

Fig 3.13 Knee bar.

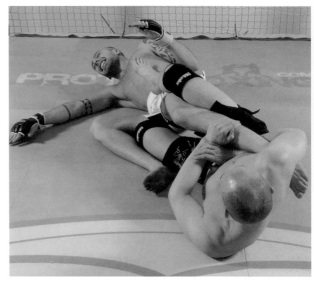

Fig 3.14 Leg lock.

In MMA there are a variety of hold-down chokes, arm locks, leg locks and wrist locks. When applied, the opponent has the option to concede by tapping out.

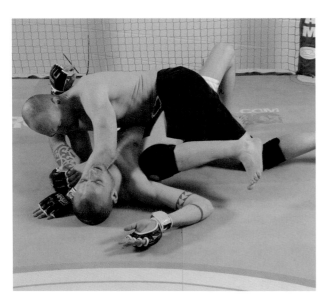

Fig 3.15 Pinning technique – knee to body.

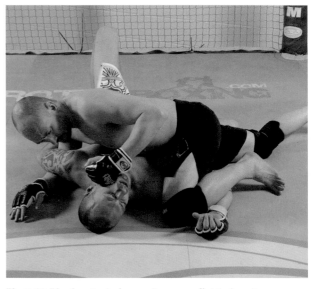

Fig 3.16 Pinning technique – hammer fist to head.

MMA ground fighting techniques differ to other ground fighting martial arts such as Brazilian jiu-jitsu because striking is allowed when on the ground.

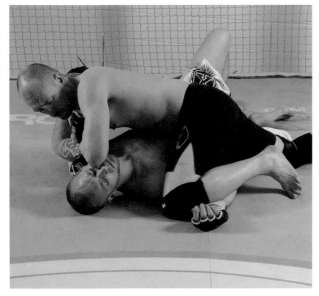

Fig 3.17 Ground fighting technique – elbowing.

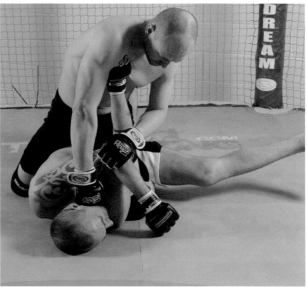

Fig 3.18 Ground fighting technique – punch.

Boxing and kicking techniques have also been adapted for the MMA arena as the stances would otherwise be too upright and the lead foot too far forward, leaving the fighter open to takedowns and kicks to the knee and thighs.

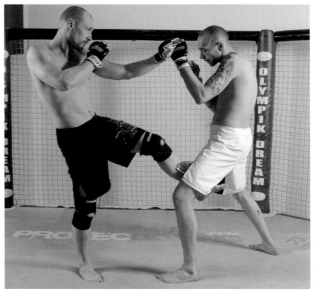

Fig 3.19 A kick to the upper knee is executed at a 45-degree angle, making it harder to defend against.

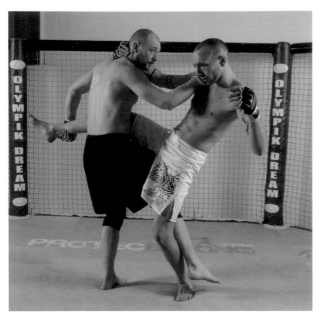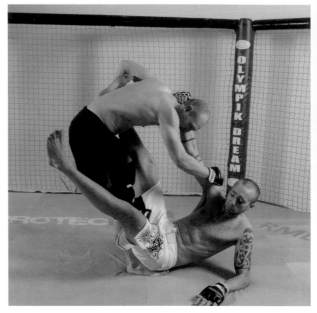

Fig 3.20 Kicking techniques executed incorrectly can result in a takedown.

Techniques and skills used and the concept behind them

The concept of MMA is very similar to that of Jeet Kune Do (JKD), which promotes the use of only those techniques that are useful and suited to each individual fighter, thus creating different but intelligent fighting styles. However, it is also advisable to train to improve any weaknesses. JKD was created by Bruce Lee in 1967.

The techniques covered by MMA fighters are:

- **Stand-up**: Taken from boxing, kick-boxing, Thai boxing and similar styles because they improve footwork due to the variety of striking techniques such as punching, kicking, kneeing and elbowing.

- **Clinching**: Taken from wrestling, judo and similar styles because they improve clinching, takedowns and throws.

- **Ground fighting**: Taken from Brazilian jiu-jitsu, wrestling, judo and similar styles because they improve submission holds, defence against submission holds, and also improve control of an opponent on the floor.

All of the above skills are needed to become a well-rounded fighter in MMA. However, the techniques have to be modified in order to be effective in this arena.

What makes MMA special and different to other martial arts

MMA differs from other martial arts because practitioners have to be open-minded about the various techniques available. A technique from an alternative martial art can be adapted and added to their existing fighting portfolio.

MMA therefore becomes unique to each practitioner although, as mentioned above, the concept is very similar to Jeet Kune Do.

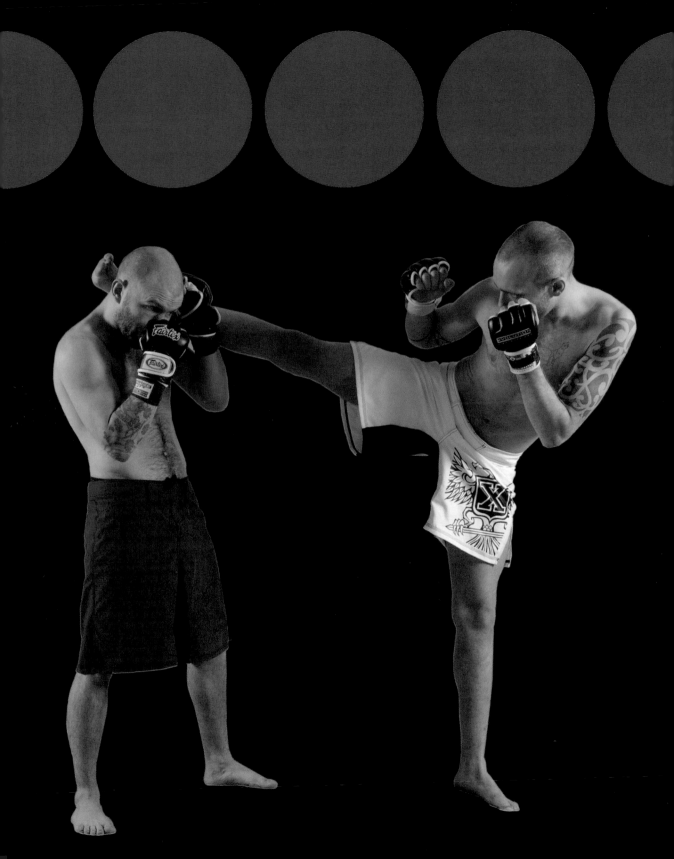

CHAPTER **FOUR**
Fighting strategies

The attraction of MMA lies in its range of techniques and fighting skills including kicking, punching, kneeing and elbowing strikes. Practitioners also have to be good at clinching, wrestling and groundwork. Any weaknesses shown in these areas will quickly be exploited by an opponent. Fitness is important too, as is a strong and agile mind that can formulate and execute an effective strategy to defeat the opponent while competing.

The main focus of MMA is the exploitation of an opponent's weaknesses combined with the imposition of one's own strengths. An effective fighter is one who can adapt in this way, but who also minimises their own weaknesses while maximising their strengths. The fighter's choice to fight standing or on the ground will be dictated by the opponent's background.

The concept of combining fighting styles was first pioneered by Bruce Lee. He believed that combining other styles into his concept and philosophy, which he called Jeet Kune Do, would give the fighter an advantage. He also felt that a good fighter should be able to adapt to the opponent's fighting style, which is also true for Mixed Martial Arts. Bruce Lee's concept was recognised by UFC president Dana White, who called Bruce Lee 'the father of Mixed Martial Arts'.

In the first MMA contests different styles competed against each other in order to see which had the advantage in a realistic confrontation, and it was not uncommon to see boxers fighting judo or karate martial artists. As the sport continued to develop, most MMA fighters trained in a wide range of styles. Today the successful MMA fighter understands the importance of being experienced in different disciplines.

MMA fighters often train in elements of boxing, kick-boxing and Thai boxing to enhance their punching, kneeing, elbowing and kicking skills. The takedown, clinching and throwing techniques are gained by training in sambo, judo and wrestling. To gain skills in submission holds and ground work, fighters use Brazilian jiu-jitsu, judo, sambo, pankration and wrestling.

Although modern MMA fighters train in a variety of styles and strategies, they often have a preference for what has proved successful for them in competitions, and examples are discussed in this chapter.

Sprawl and brawl

A strategy used by fighters whose strengths are in striking techniques and stand-up fighting. These fighters try to keep the fight standing and avoid being taken down by developing appropriate defence techniques. They specialise in knockout kicks, punches, knees and elbows. In case they do end up on the ground, most of these fighters are trained in submission wrestling. If a fighter who prefers the sprawl and brawl strategy is taken to the ground, they try to stall their opponent until the referee brings the fight back to standing. Alternatively, they try to escape from their opponent and return to their feet.

This strategy is often used by fighters such as Mirko Cro Cop or Chuck Liddell.

Clinch fighting

A strategy involving holding an opponent in a clinch and either going for a takedown or applying elbow/knee strikes, punches or stomps. Fighters with a strong wrestling or Muay Thai (Thai boxing) background are keen on this style, which can be devastating for an opponent. The clinch is used to prevent the opponent from moving away and to keep them within range for strikes and takedowns. The clinch can also be used as a defence against strikes and takedowns.

In the professional arena, Randy Couture and Anderson Silva are good examples of fighters who use this strategy to their advantage.

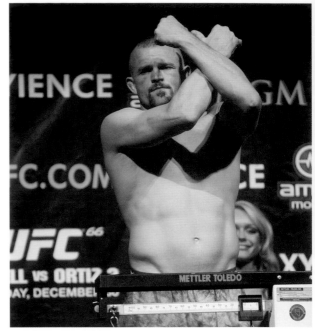

Fig 4.1 Chuck Liddell.

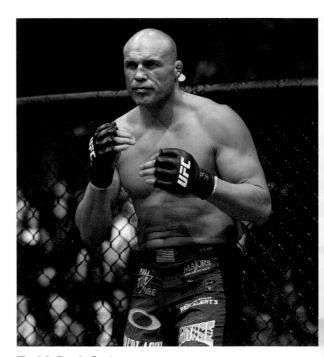

Fig 4.2 Randy Couture.

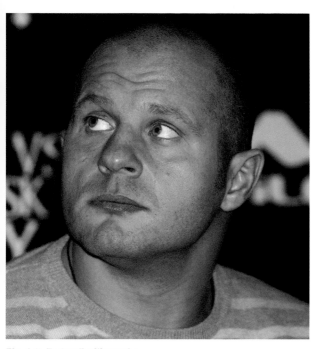

Fig 4.3 Fedor Emilianenko

Submission grappling

A fighter applying the submission grappling strategy takes their opponent to the ground with a throw or takedown to achieve a dominant position and apply a submission hold. Fighters using this strategy do so because they prefer working on the ground and feel comfortable with the variety of ground fighting positions.

Fighters known to be effective in applying this strategy are Royce Gracie and Fedor Emelianenko.

Ground and pound

A ground fighting strategy which takes the opponent to the ground with takedowns or throws. Once there, the fighter gets on top of them to gain the dominant position and then pummels them with punches and elbows until they are knocked out or submit. This strategy has proved that good striking techniques can also be effective on the ground when maintaining a grappling position.

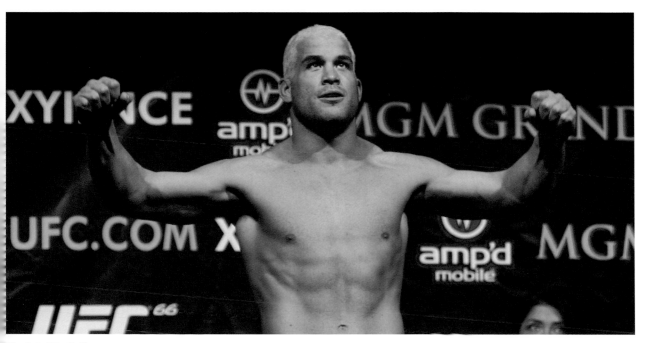

Fig 4.4 Tito Ortiz

The UFC and PRIDE grand prix champion Mark Coleman was one of the first fighters to prove the effectiveness of this strategy. Randy Couture and Tito Ortiz have also shown its merit and it has become part of MMA training.

Lay and pray

The strategy of lay and pray involves the fighter taking the opponent to the ground, gaining a dominant or neutral position and hoping that a victory can be claimed by pinning them there. The tempo and action are taken out of the fight, which is stalled in the hope that it can be won by the judge's decision rather than a knockout or submission. This strategy can be favoured by wrestlers as they have takedown skills, but little experience in submission grappling or ground and pound. Lay and pray is used by fighters who are not as capable on the ground.

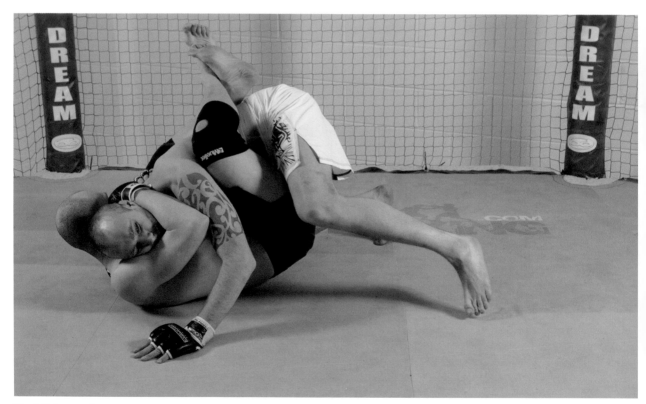

Fig 4.5 Lay and pray

Multiple strategies (hybrid styles)

This term is used to describe fighters who use a wide range of strategies to gain victory. They are well trained in striking, submission techniques and ground and pound. Most fighters rely on a limited base of strengths and do not have this wide range. As such, they must always defend against their weaknesses.

Good examples of fighters applying multiple strategies are B J Penn and Fedor Emelianenko.

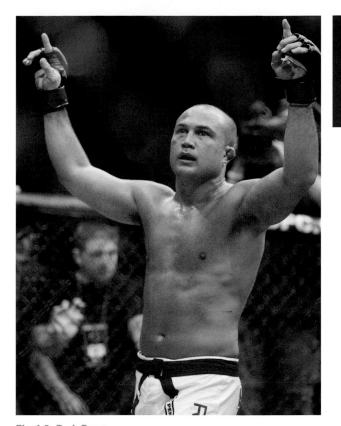

Fig 4.6 B. J. Penn

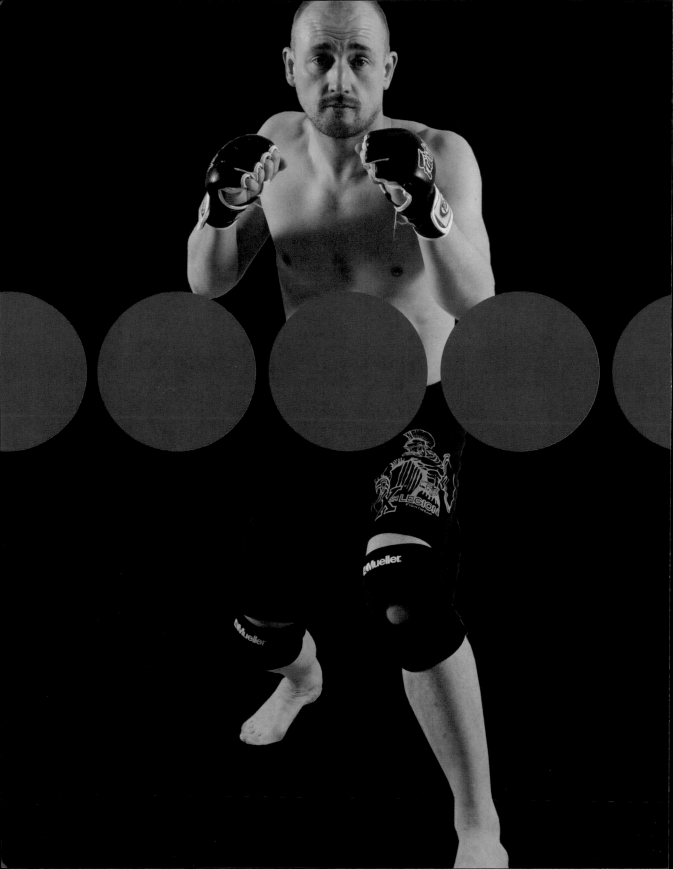

CHAPTER **FIVE**
Stances

Stances and footwork are very important in MMA as they allow for quick transitions into strikes, grapples, sprawls, shoots and takedowns at all ranges.

Balance is also important, so the stance should not be too wide or too narrow and the feet should ideally be shoulder width apart. The stance should be re-established as often as possible when moving around. This also helps prevent the legs from crossing and the stance from becoming too spread.

Standard stance

The standard stance is used when moving around the fighting area because it allows for fast movement and easy strikes. The shoulders should be square to the opponent and the hips slightly angled with one leg in front of the other. This reduces the risk of being taken down: the legs are not beside each other and it is possible to crouch down further.

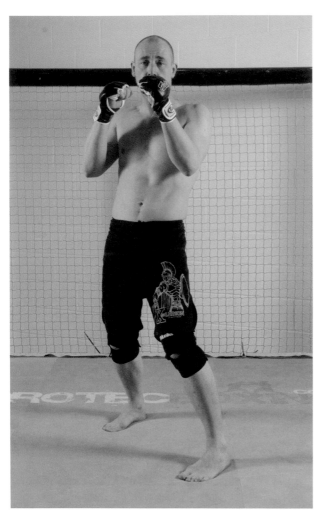

Fig 5.1 The standard boxing, kick-boxing and Thai boxing stance with the hips and feet facing the opponent and the shoulders at an angle.

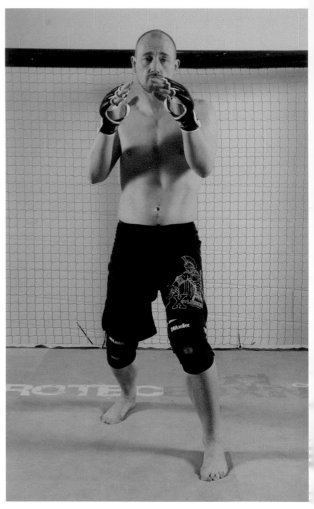

Fig 5.2 The standard MMA stance, with the shoulders square to the opponent, the hips angled and one foot behind the other. The guard is up to protect the face and ribs, and the knees are slightly bent. This stance also makes it easier to assume a crouched stance.

Crouched stance

The crouched stance is the same as the standard stance, only lower and with the upper body bent forward to align the head with the front leg. This stance is used in preparation for a takedown or to defend against one by sprawling. It can also be used as a feint before returning to the standard stance and striking if an opening has been created.

A common error with the crouched stance is to lean forward without lowering the body. This hinders movement and presents the opponent with an easier target to strike.

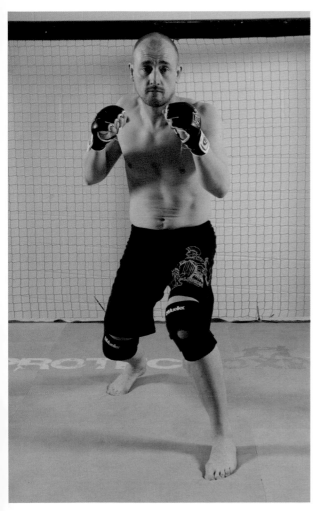

Fig 5.3 The standard MMA stance.

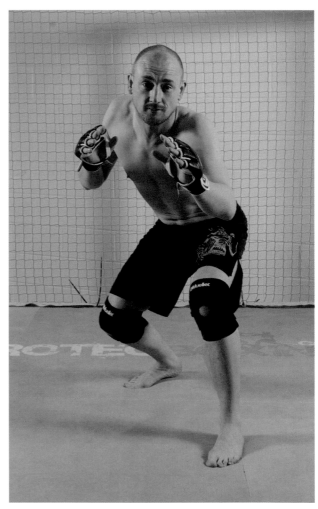

Fig 5.4 The crouched MMA stance. Knees are bent and the posture is lower than the standard MMA stance. The guard is up to protect the face and ribs.

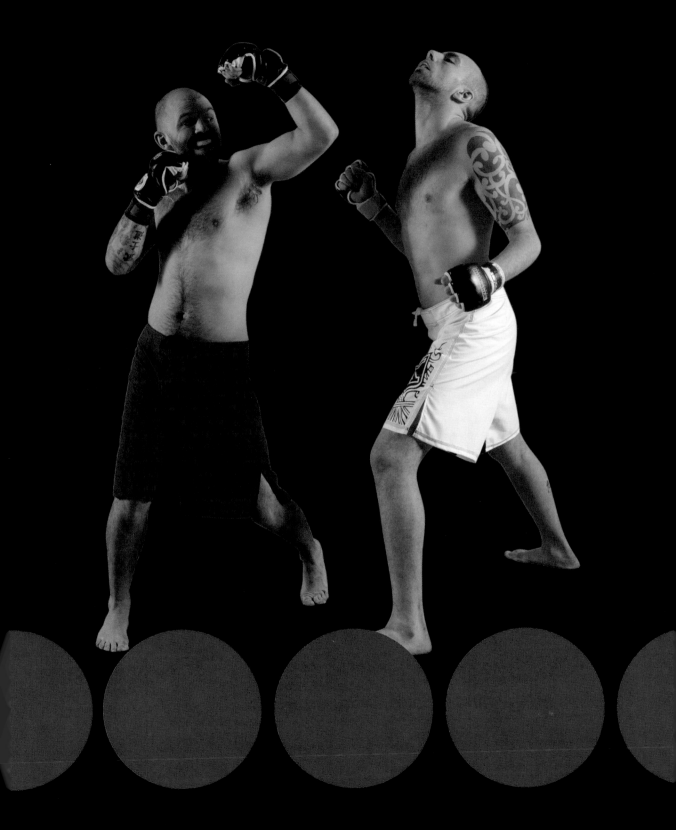

CHAPTER **SIX**
Strikes

In MMA there are hundreds of different types of strikes, the most common of which have been included here. Basic principles apply to all and it is important to understand these when competing in a full contact sport.

Punches

Every punch should be delivered with the whole body movement as this improves effectiveness. Combinations of punches are a useful way to distract an opponent. Because of the speed of the sequence of individual strikes that make up a combination, they are also difficult to defend against. Possible opportunities created might include openings for takedowns or a kick to the torso as the opponent protects their head with their hands. Alternatively, punches can be used to keep an opponent away or as an attacking sequence to knock them out.

Key principles

- Relax and don't tense up.

- Use the whole body by turning the hips into the punch.

- Keep the chin tucked under.

- Keep the non-punching hand close to the face to protect against counter-attacks.

- Use combinations of punches as they are more effective.

- After each punch, quickly return to the starting position.

THE JAB

Although the jab is not the most powerful punch, it is considered to be one of the most important because it can help keep an opponent away. It can also be used to set up other striking combinations or takedowns, and to defend against attacks.

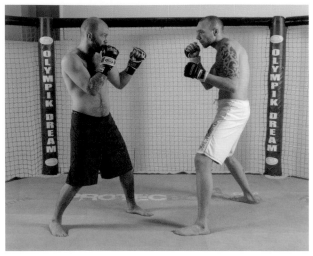

Fig 6.1 The fighting stance, with the jab hand in front and the non-punching hand protecting the face.

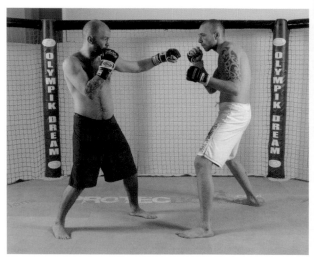

Fig 6.2 The jab partly executed. The hip is turned into the punch. The hand starts to turn so the palm will be facing downwards when the punch is executed.

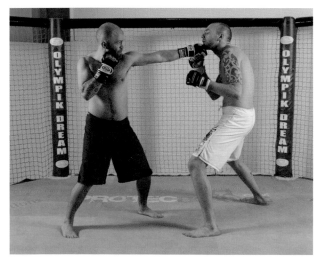

Fig 6.3 The jab executed. The hand is fully turned, with the palm facing downwards and the chin tucked behind the shoulder of the punching hand. The non-punching hand is tight against the face to protect against counter-attacks. The hip is turned into the jab to generate more power.

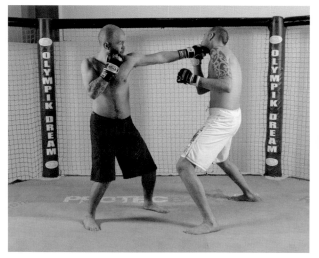

Fig 6.4 To generate more power, a small step forward can be made on the same side as the punching hand.

THE CROSS

The right cross, also known as the straight right, is one of the most powerful knockout punches and can be used to attack or counter-attack. The main benefit of using this strike as a counter-attack is the additional power gained by the combination of the opponent's body weight coming forward to attack, with the cross action of the punch.

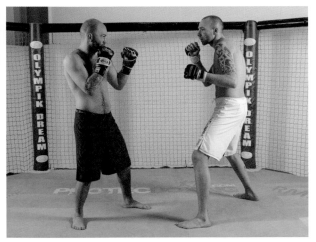

Fig 6.5 The fighting stance, with the non-punching hand in front and the other protecting the face.

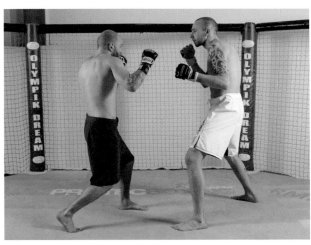

Fig 6.6 The cross partially executed. The hip is turned into the cross and the hand starts to turn so that the palm will face downwards when the punch is executed.

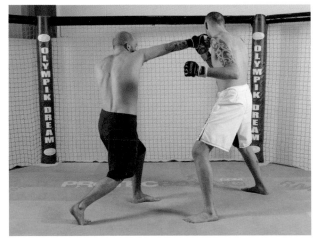

Fig 6.7 The cross executed. The punching hand is fully rotated with the palm facing downwards. The chin is tucked behind the shoulder of the punching hand and the non-punching hand is tight to the face to protect against counter-attacks. The hip is turned into the cross and the rear foot pivots to put the body weight behind the punch.

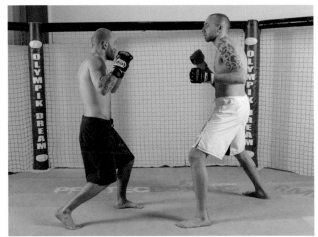

Fig 6.8 More power can be generated by using a small step forward with the opposite leg to the punching hand. When the leg touches the ground, pivot the rear leg to put the body weight behind the punch.

THE HOOK

When applied correctly, the hook can be a knockout punch, especially when all of the body weight is put behind it by rotating the hips. It is also a difficult punch to block as the hand follows the line of an arch. The hook can be used to attack, counter-attack or as a transition for a takedown.

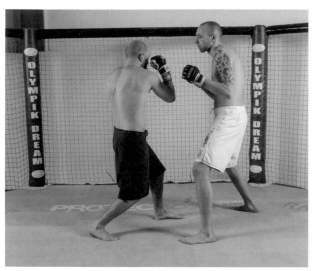

Fig 6.9 The fighting stance before the hook.

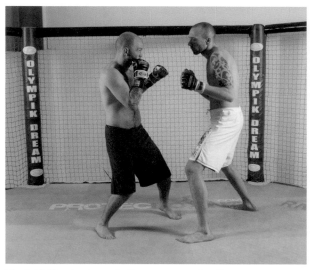

Fig 6.10 The hook partially executed. The fist is turned with the palm facing downwards and the arm is at an angle of at least 90 degrees.

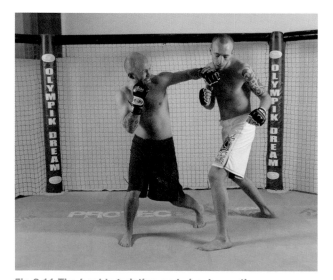

Fig 6.11 The hook's twisting and circular motion.

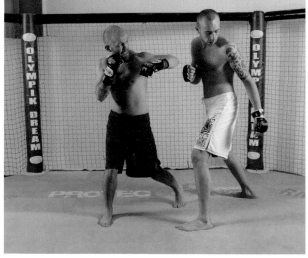

Fig 6.12 The end position. The hook's power is increased by the circular motion of the body.

THE UPPERCUT

The uppercut is a powerful knockout strike used at close proximity and usually aimed at the chin, floating ribs or solar plexus. Power is generated from the upward linear motion created by the turning of the hips, legs and shoulders.

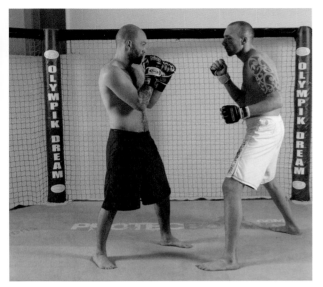

Fig 6.13 The fighting stance before the uppercut.

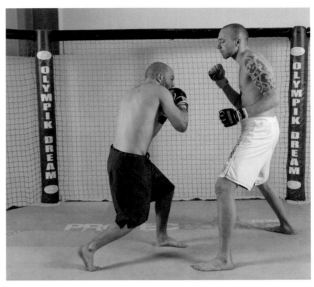

Fig 6.14 Dropping down into a crouched position with the guard up.

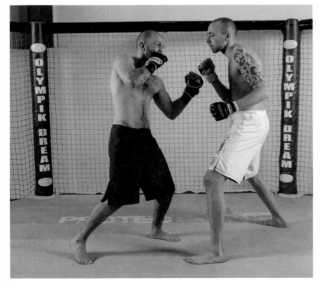

Fig 6.15 Maintaining the crouch, the palm of the punching fist is turned towards the body. The body weight is put behind the punch by twisting the body in the direction of the punch.

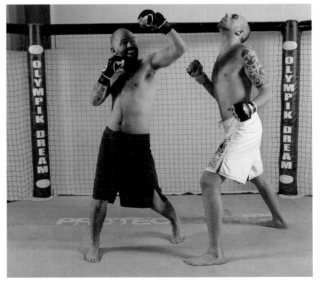

Fig 6.16 While the body is turning, the weight is transferred on to the leg on the same side as the punching arm and directs the motion upward.

41

THE OVERHAND

The overhand right is a hybrid technique combining elements of the hook and right cross to generate an effective knockout punch, or to get past an opponent's defences. The motion of the overhand is forward and slightly curved.

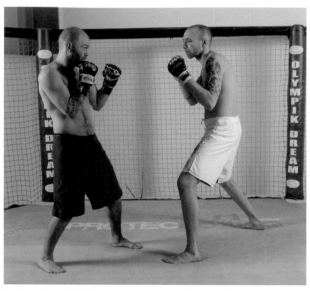

Fig 6.17 The fighting stance before the overhand.

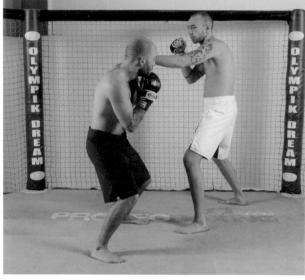

Fig 6.18 A short step forward and to the left is taken as the right hand is brought over the opponent's head.

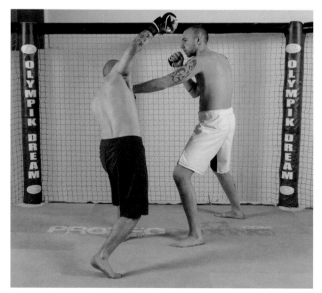

Fig 6.19 The arm is arched over the opponent's defence and the body is turned anti-clockwise to bring the fist in closer.

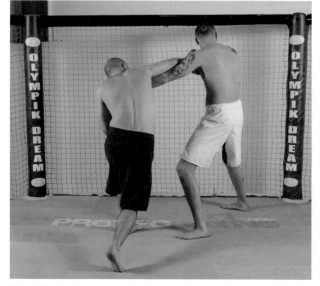

Fig 6.20 As the punch is placed, the arm is extended, the weight is brought forward, and the rear foot pivots.

THE SPINNING BACK FIST

The spinning back fist is a remarkable and powerful punch that can often surprise an opponent. The whipping motion is generated by bending the elbow of the striking arm and timing the contact to occur while the body is still turning.

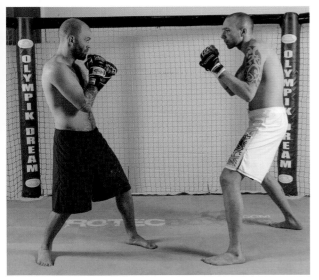

Fig 6.21 The fighting stance before the spinning back fist.

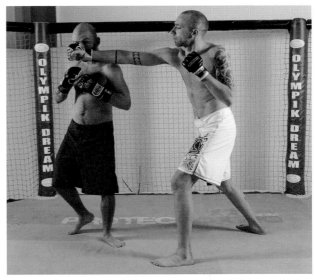

Fig 6.22 The striking arm is bent and the body is spun as fast as possible anticlockwise on the left foot.

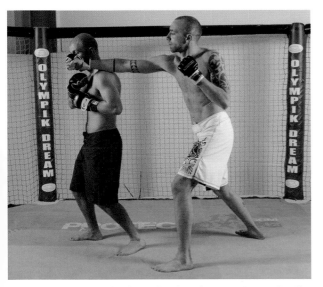

Fig 6.23 While spinning, the head turns towards the opponent and the punch is placed.

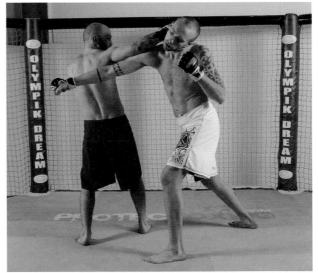

Fig 6.24 The punch is placed using the side of the fist, which is whipped out by straightening the arm combining with the power of the spin.

Elbow strikes

The elbow strike is a very powerful technique that can knock out an opponent when executed correctly. Power is generated by a circular motion of the elbow and a twisting action of the body. It can be used to attack or counter-attack when standing or on the ground and is difficult to block.

Key principles

■ Relax and don't tense up.

■ Use the whole body by turning into the strike.

■ Keep the non-striking arm over the face to guard against counter-attacks.

■ Aim through the opponent as this generates more power.

■ After each strike, quickly return to the starting position.

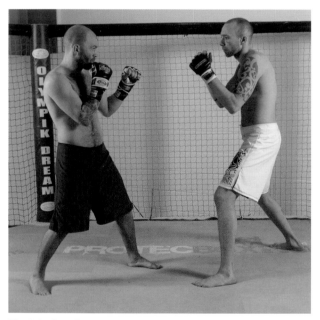

Fig 6.25 The fighting stance before the elbow strike.

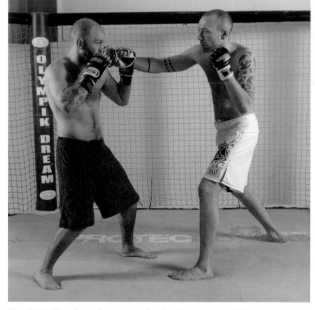

Fig 6.26 The face is covered with the non-striking hand and the elbowing arm is ready at a 45-degree angle.

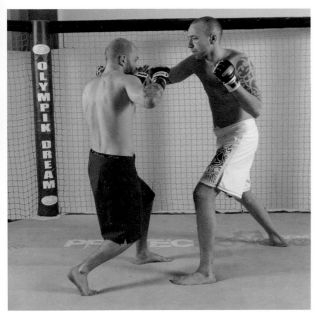 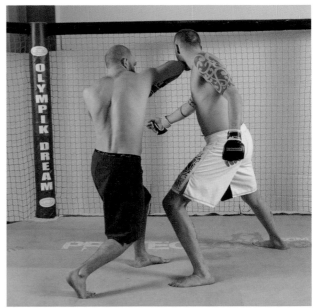

Fig 6.27 The elbow travels horizontally towards the opponent with the whole body weight behind it, achieved by pivoting on the foot that is on the same side as the striking elbow.

Fig 6.28 The executed elbow, with pivoted feet and turned body.

THE UPWARD ELBOW STRIKE

The upward elbow strike follows the same line and principles as the uppercut. Power is generated by the upward linear motion of the elbow combined with the force created by turning the hips, legs and shoulders. It is an excellent method of getting past an opponent's defences and can also knock them out when placed on their chin. However, it is a versatile technique that can be used in many situations.

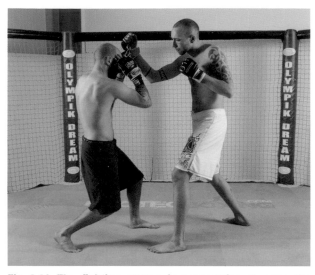

Fig 6.29 The fighting stance in preparation to pass the opponent's defences.

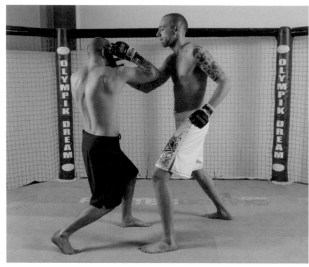

Fig 6.30 The face is covered with the non-striking hand and the elbowing arm is ready at a 45-degree angle.

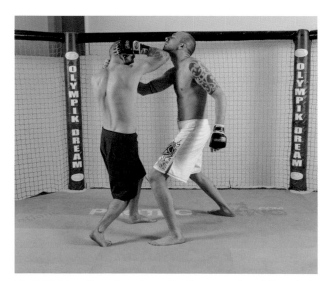

Fig 6.31 The elbow travels vertically upward and the whole body is turned into the movement by pivoting on the foot that is on the same side as the striking elbow.

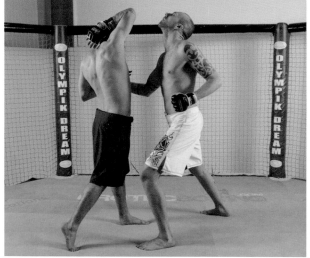

Fig 6.32 The executed elbow strike, with pivoted feet and turned body.

Punching and elbowing on the ground

Ground and pound is a famous MMA technique, in which the opponent can be punched or elbowed while on the floor. This can continue until the opponent is knocked out or submits by tapping out. For the technique to be effective the fighter needs to be upright and not restricted by the opponent.

Figures 6.33 and 6.34 show how the fighter can generate more power with an upright position and freedom of space. The advantage has been given away by the opponent as they have not controlled the fighter's head.

In figure 6.35 the fighter controls their opponent's head and restricts them from freely punching or elbowing. Any strikes the opponent could apply would have reduced power.

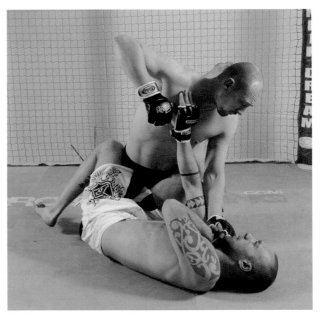

Fig 6.33 An upright position generates more power for a punch.

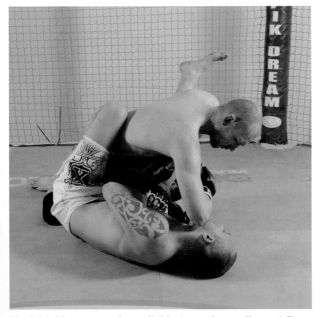

Fig 6.34 More power is available to apply an elbow strike.

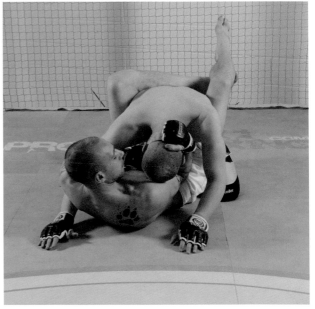

Fig 6.35 The fighter controls their opponent's head and restricts their movement.

Kicks

A correctly delivered kick can be three times more powerful than a punch and is generated by a quick flick of the hips just before impact. Mirko Filipovic, or 'Cro Cop', proved how effective this can be for knockouts.

Key principles

- ■ Relax and don't tense up.

- ■ Use the whole body movement by turning the hip into the kick.

- ■ The heel of the non-kicking leg should point towards the opponent when a kick is executed.

- ■ Keep the guard up while kicking.

- ■ Use combinations, as these are more effective.

- ■ After each kick, quickly return to the starting position.

THE ROUNDHOUSE KICK

The roundhouse kick is probably the most frequently used kicking technique in MMA and can result in knockouts. Kicks can be made to any part of the opponent's body, with impact being made with either the top of the foot or the shin. The same key principles apply to all kicking variations, which can be performed from either the front or back leg as an attacking, defensive or counter-attacking technique.

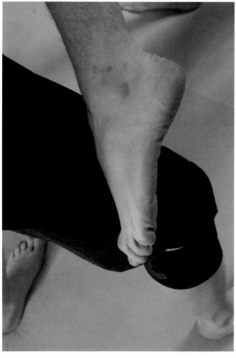

Fig 6.36 The top of the foot striking area.

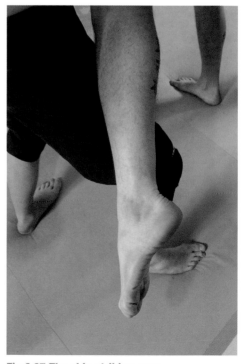

Fig 6.37 The shin striking area.

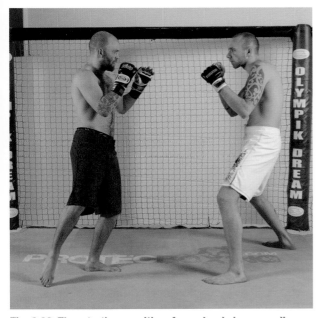

Fig 6.38 The starting position for a back-leg roundhouse kick, with the majority of the weight on the front leg.

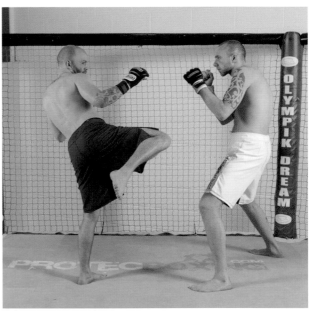

Fig 6.39 The kicking leg is prepared, or chambered, and the heel of the non-kicking leg is pointing towards the opponent.

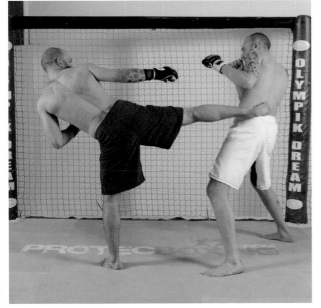

Fig 6.40 The kick is snapped out and the hip is turned in just before impact to generate more power.

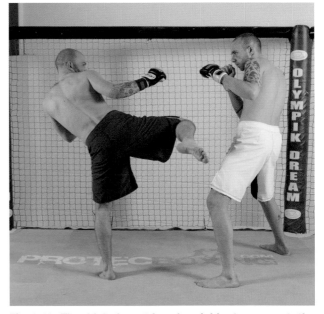

Fig 6.41 The kick is retrieved quickly to prevent the opponent from grabbing the leg. Also, when the fighter has both feet on the ground he is more mobile.

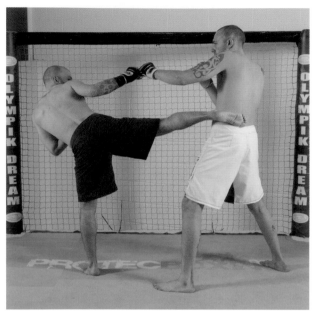

Fig 6.42 To make it more difficult for the opponent to catch the leg, the kick can travel up at a 45-degree angle.

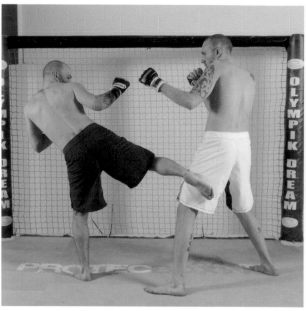

Fig 6.43 This also applies to low kicks to the thigh and when applied regularly can wear an opponent down.

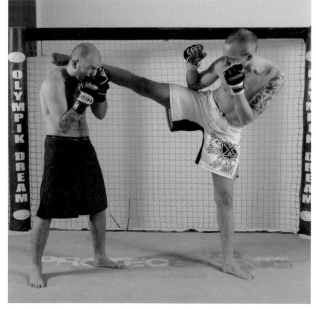

Fig 6.44 A roundhouse kick to the head is a very effective knockout technique requiring good flexibility.

THE SIDE KICK

Side kicks are commonly deployed for low or midsection strikes and use either the heel or the outside of the foot. They can be performed from the front or back leg and used as an attacking or counter-attacking technique.

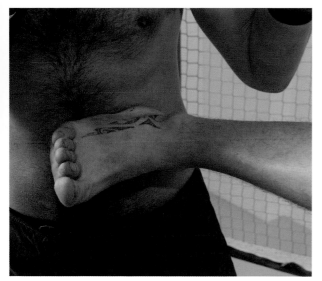

Fig 6.45 The heel striking area.

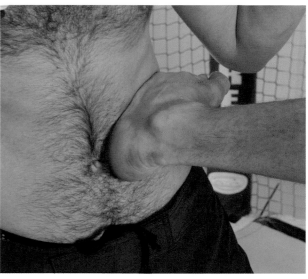

Fig 6.46 The outside of the foot striking area.

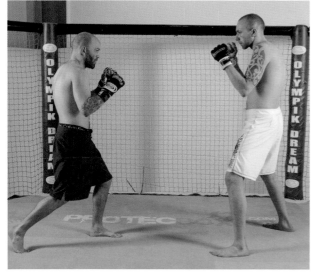

Fig 6.47 The starting position for a back-leg side kick, with most of the weight on the front leg.

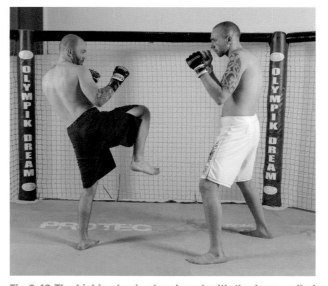

Fig 6.48 The kicking leg is chambered with the knee pulled towards the chest. The heel of the non-kicking leg points towards the opponent.

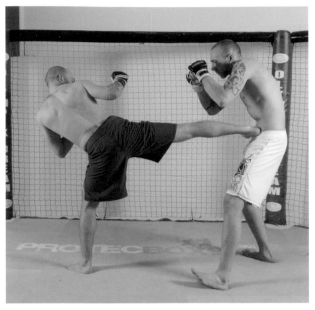

Fig 6.49 The kick is snapped out and the hip is rotated forward just before impact as this generates more power. The toes of the kicking leg point downwards.

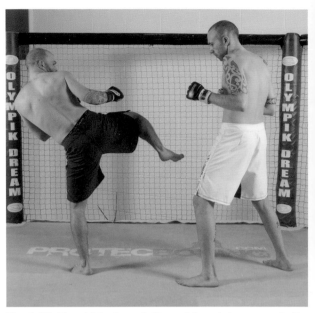

Fig 6.50 The kick is quickly retrieved to prevent the opponent from grabbing the leg. Also, when the fighter has both feet on the ground he is more mobile.

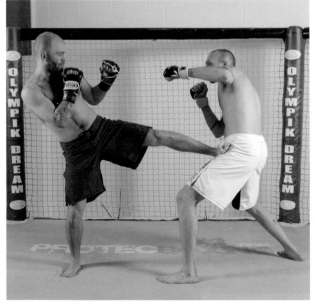

Fig 6.51 The side kick can be used to stop an opponent's attack by kicking to the thigh with the front leg.

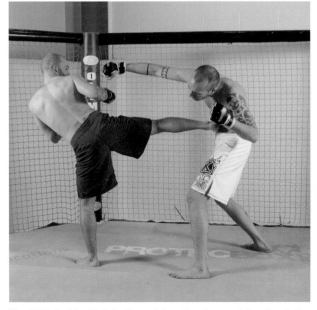

Fig 6.52 A side kick to the midsection is used to attack the opponent and to bridge the gap so other techniques or takedowns can be applied.

THE FRONT KICK

A front kick can be applied to all areas of the opponent's body and strikes are made using the ball or sole of the foot. The kick can be performed using the front or back leg as either an attacking or counter-attacking technique. It is very simple, but fast and effective.

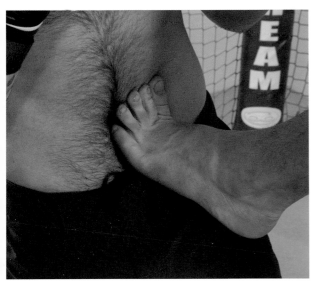

Fig 6.53 The ball of the foot striking area.

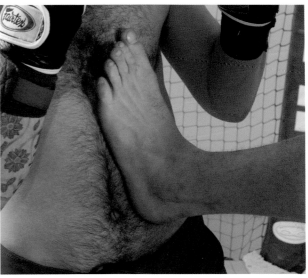

Fig 6.54 The sole of the foot striking area.

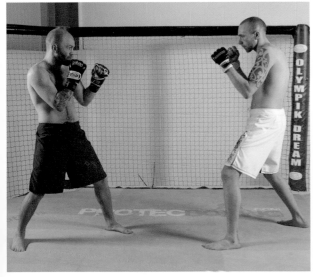

Fig 6.55 The fighting stance. A front kick performed with the back leg requires the majority of the weight to be on the non-kicking leg.

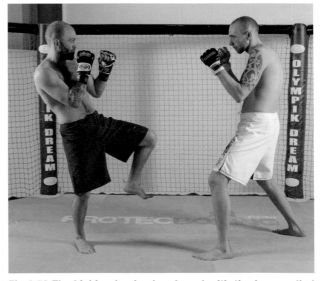

Fig 6.56 The kicking leg is chambered with the knee pulled vertically towards the chest.

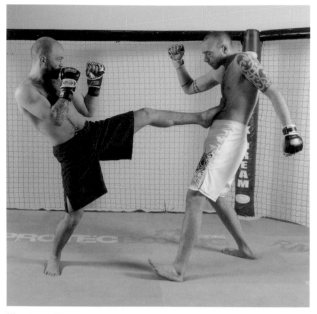

Fig 6.57 The toes are pulled back and the foot snapped forward. The hip is also pushed forward to add power.

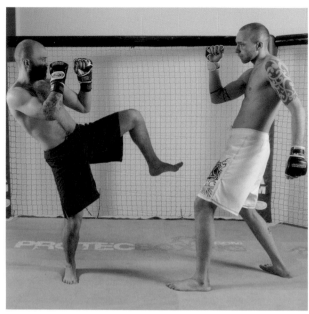

Fig 6.58 The kicking foot is snapped back and placed either in front or behind the other leg.

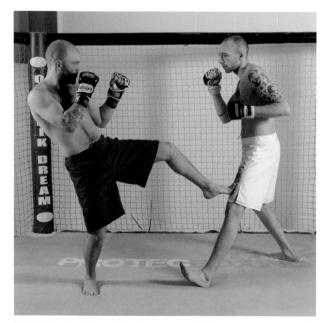

Fig 6.59 The front kick can be used to stop an opponent's attack. Here the front leg is used to kick the opponent's upper knee.

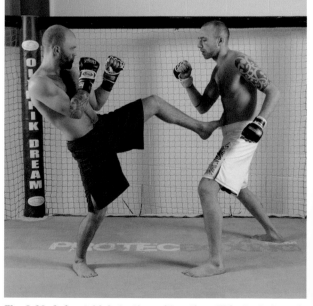

Fig 6.60 A front kick to the midsection. This technique is used to attack the opponent and bridge the gap so it can be followed up with other attacking techniques or a takedown.

THE SPINNING HOOK KICK

The spinning hook kick is normally used to strike the opponent's head. When performed and timed correctly, it can result in a knockout. The heel of the foot is used for the strike, which is normally performed with the back leg. It is also a very good move to use to defend against an attacking opponent.

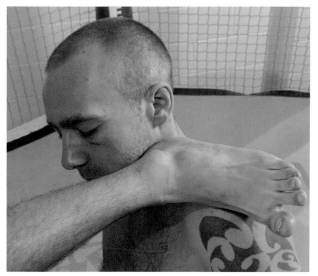

Fig 6.61 The heel striking area.

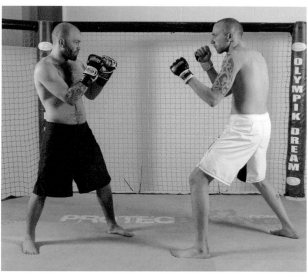

Fig 6.62 In the fighting stance the weight is evenly distributed. The fighter then pivots on both feet so their back and heels face the opponent as in figure 6.63.

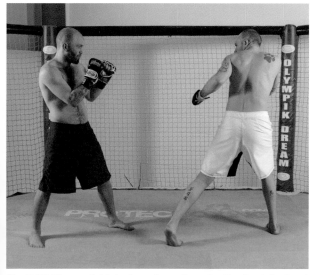

Fig 6.63 The weight is transferred on to the foot furthest from the opponent and the head turns towards them.

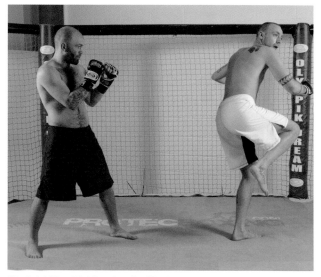

Fig 6.64 The kicking leg is lifted and chambered.

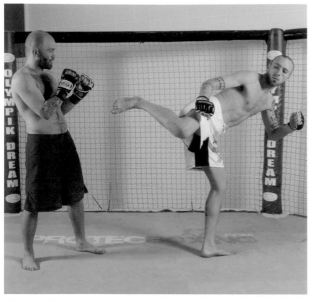

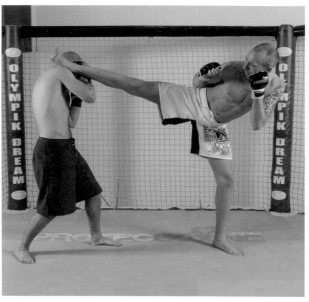

Fig 6.65 The foot is snapped out fast, travelling in an arc to a point past the opponent's head.

Fig 6.66 The executed kick against the opponent's head.

OTHER KICKS

Many other kicks can be performed depending on the fighter's skill and also whether the opponent is on the ground or standing.

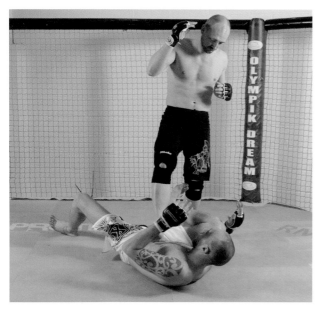

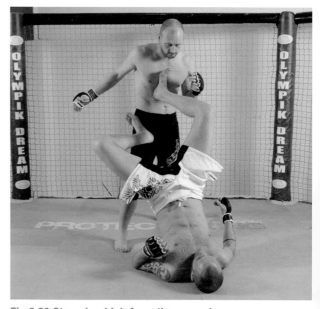

Fig 6.67 Downward stomp kick.

Fig 6.68 Stomping kick from the ground.

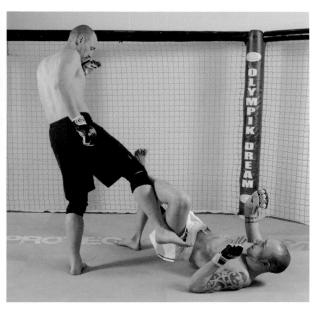

Fig 6.69 Soccer kick.

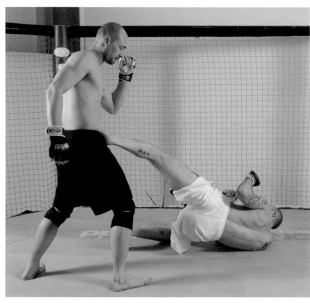

Fig 6.70 Side push kick.

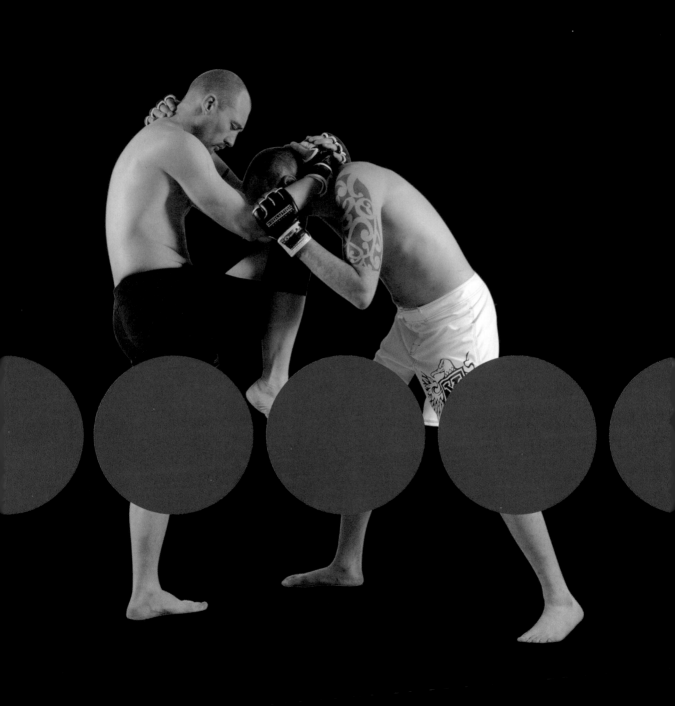

CHAPTER SEVEN
Stand-up grappling

Stand-up grappling techniques are very important in MMA and an advantage is gained by perfecting them. Once mastered, other techniques can be combined with the grapple, such as strikes with knees and elbows, or punches and takedowns.

The clinch

The clinch is used in many other martial arts with the best examples coming from Muay Thai and wrestling. In wrestling the clinch focuses on hip and body control, and in Muay Thai it focuses on head control. Another method is the dirty boxing clinch, which involves holding the opponent's head with one arm, pushing and pulling them off balance and then delivering punches to the head and body.

The Muay Thai clinch

The Muay Thai clinch focuses on controlling the opponent's head, then using this control to push and pull them off balance and to apply punches and knee and elbow strikes.

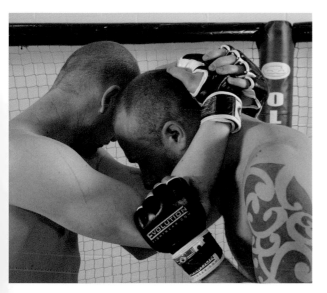

Fig 7.1 The opponent's head is held tightly in the Muay Thai clinch, with the hands lying unlinked on top of each other.

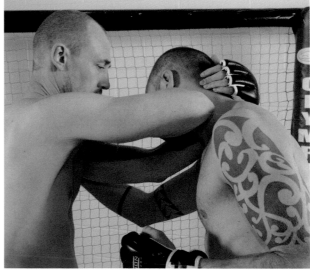

Fig 7.2 An elbow strike thrown from the clinch.

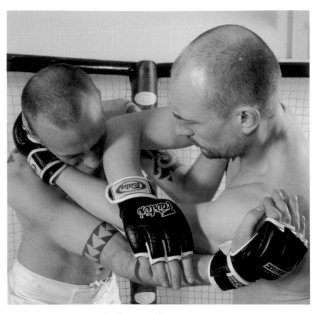

Fig 7.3 An executed elbow strike.

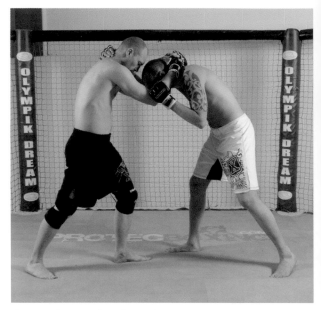

Fig 7.4 Preparation for a knee strike to the head. It is important for the opponent's head to be lowered and this is achieved by the fighter jumping back with the kneeing leg to create the desired space and lower stance.

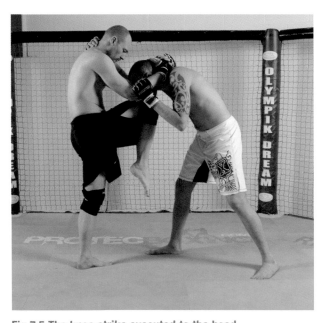

Fig 7.5 The knee strike executed to the head.

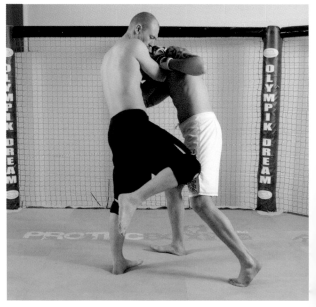

Fig 7.6 A knee strike executed from the side for targeting the short ribs or the thighs.

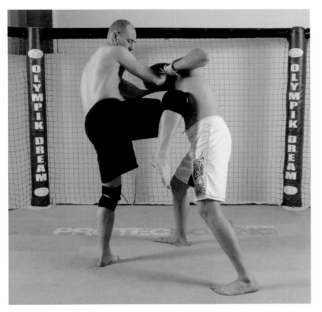

Fig 7.7 A knee strike executed from the side to the short rib. Before executing, the fighter pulls the opponent's head to the side to expose the rib.

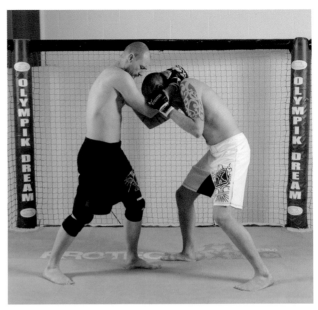

Fig 7.8 The opponent straightens up to prevent their head from being pulled down.

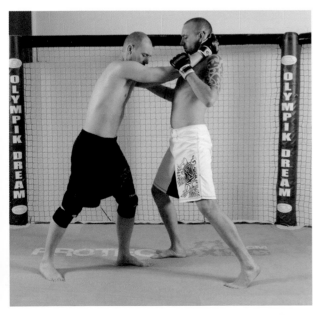

Fig 7.9 The opponent's resistance results in the fighter letting go of the Muay Thai clinch.

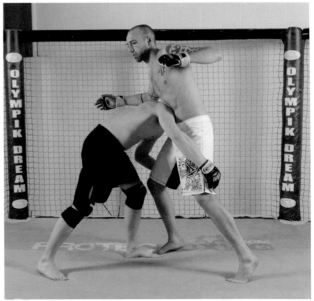

Fig 7.10 However, the fighter capitalises on their opponent's vulnerable upright position by shooting in for a takedown.

Escaping the Muay Thai clinch

The Muay Thai clinch is very powerful because once in place other techniques can be applied to make the opponent extremely vulnerable. It is therefore important to be able to quickly counteract it.

ESCAPE 1

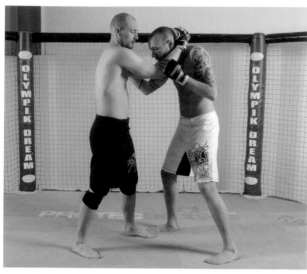

Fig 7.11 The Muay Thai clinch.

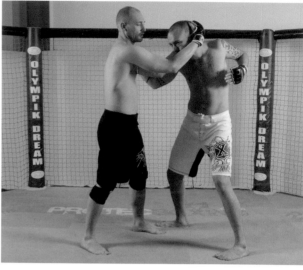

Fig 7.12 The clinched fighter tries to get inside the clinch by bringing one arm through.

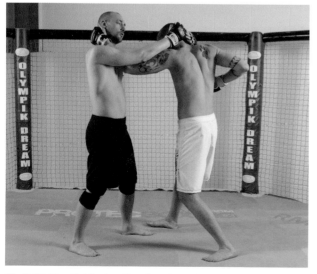

Fig 7.13 The fighter's other hand pushes through inside the opponent's arms.

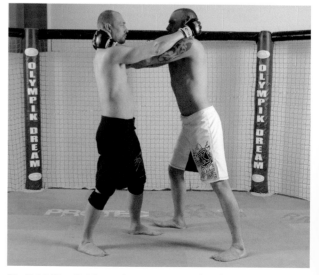

Fig 7.14 The fighter gains a secure grip of their opponent's head. The fighter now has the advantage.

ESCAPE 2

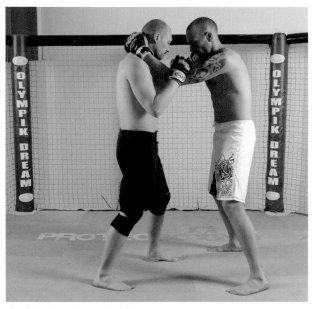

Fig 7.15 The Muay Thai clinch

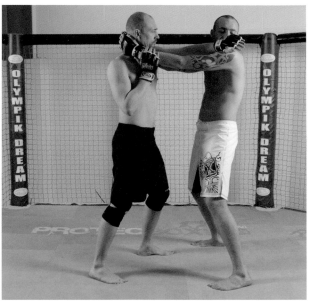

Fig 7.16 The clinched fighter puts their arm over their opponent's to push back their head. This action reduces the opponent's grip and generates a gap.

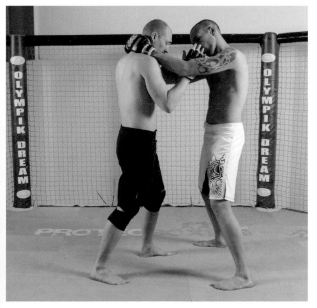

Fig 7.17 The fighter's other hand follows into the gap.

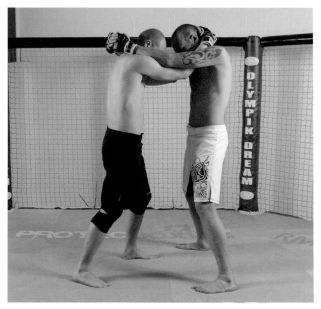

Fig 7.18 The dominant clinch.

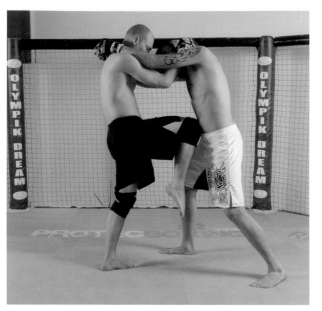 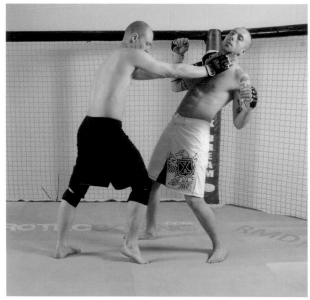

Fig 7.19 The clinching fighter applies a knee to the opponent's body to weaken him.

Fig 7.20 The fighter straightens both arms to push their opponent's head back in order to escape.

The wrestling clinch

The wrestling clinch focuses on controlling the opponent's torso and hips in order to take them down using a leg or body takedown or a throw. Both competitors try to get their arms under each other's in order to grab the top of the shoulders, waist or hips; this manoeuvre is also known as an *under hook*. When both arms of the fighter clinch the shoulders of the opponent, which is also known as a *double under hook*, an advantage is created because the body lock makes it easier to perform a takedown or a separation.

Many other techniques can be combined with the wresting clinch, two of which are shown here.

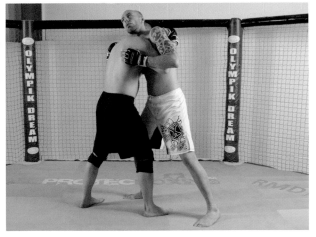

Fig 7.21 Two fighters grappling to achieve an under hook, with neither having the advantage.

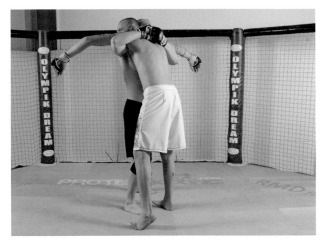

Fig 7.22 A fighter with both arms under their opponent's in a double hook. The advantage is now with the fighter.

A WRESTLE CLINCH COMBINED WITH A BODY LOCK

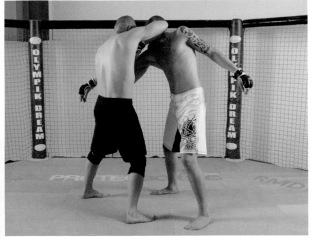

Fig 7.23 The fighter applies an elbow strike from the under hook.

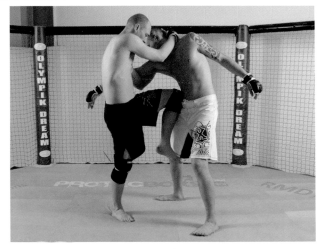

Fig 7.24 The fighter applies a knee strike from the under hook.

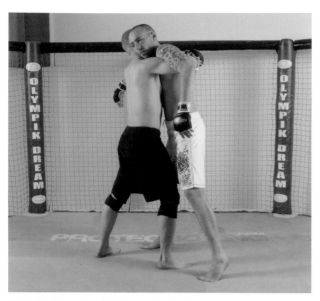

Fig 7.25 From the double under hook, the fighter moves one hand so that they are holding the wrist of their other hand behind their opponent.

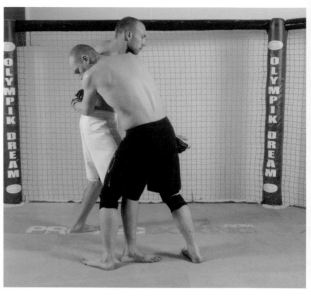

Fig 7.26 The fighter steps behind the opponent.

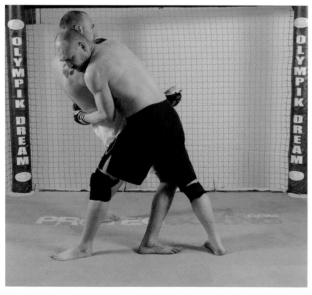

Fig 7.27 By rotating around their own axis, the fighter can trip their opponent.

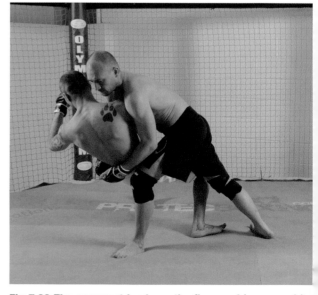

Fig 7.28 The opponent lands on the floor and is secured by the fighter using a side control.

A WRESTLE CLINCH COMBINED WITH A KNEE TO TAKEDOWN

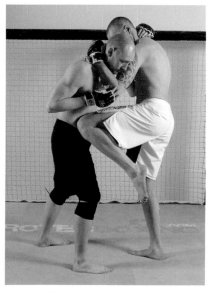

Fig 7.29 The opponent tries to get out of a clinch by using their knee.

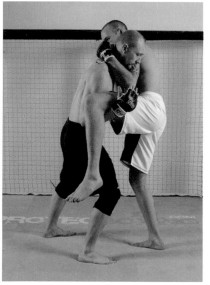

Fig 7.30 The fighter responds by getting their arm under the opponent's kneeing leg, while still maintaining their upright posture to avoid being struck by it.

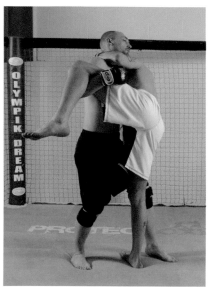

Fig 7.31 The fighter lifts the caught leg and sweeps the other foot of the opponent from under them.

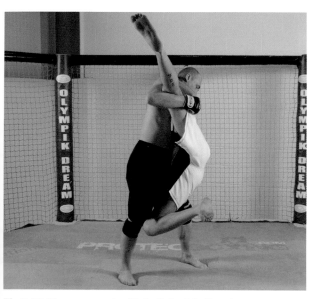

Fig 7.32 The opponent with both feet in the air.

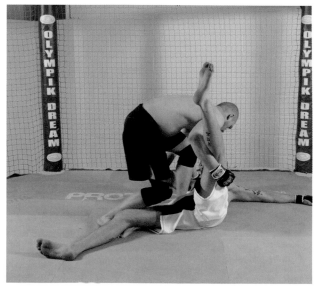

Fig 7.34 The opponent is slammed to the floor, with the fighter's arm still wrapped around their leg.

Escapes from the under hook

Because the under hook is widely used, it is important to learn how to escape from it to avoid being taken down. The best method is by lowering the hips, and therefore your centre of gravity, as this makes it harder for the opponent to execute a pick up and slam down.

ESCAPE 1 FROM THE DOUBLE UNDER HOOK

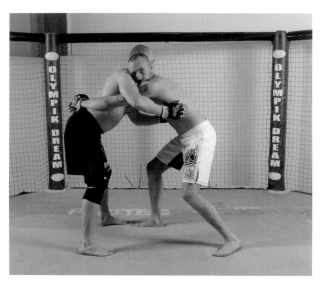

Fig 7.35 The opponent applies a double under hook and the fighter responds by lowering their hips and centre of gravity.

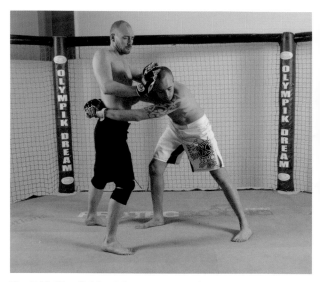

Fig 7.36 The fighter tries to escape the opponent's hold by pushing their head away with both hands. The fighter also lowers their head as this reduces the opponent's leverage for a takedown.

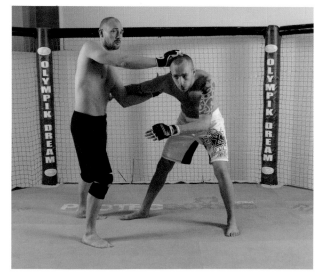

Fig 7.37 The fighter continues to move their head down to increase the separation, helped by pushing away the hip of the opponent with one hand. The fighter will then use the space created to reach through with their other arm and secure a single under hook.

ESCAPE 2 FROM THE DOUBLE UNDER HOOK

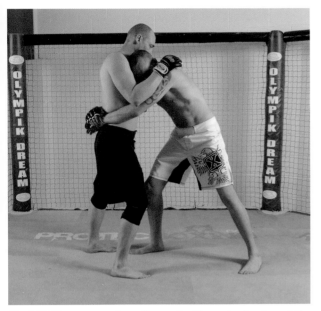

Fig 7.38 The opponent applies a double under hook and the fighter responds by lowering their hips and centre of gravity.

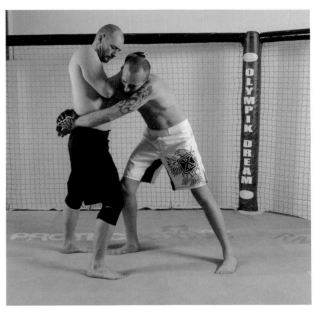

Fig 7.39 The fighter raises one elbow and wedges it between the opponent's neck and shoulder.

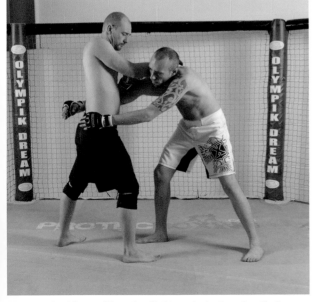

Fig 7.40 In this position the fighter starts to relax their arm, pull back and step away from the opponent.

The dirty boxing clinch

The dirty boxing clinch is used in MMA for punching and elbowing the opponent with additional momentum being created by pulling their head down as part of the strike. Pushing and pulling the opponent's head, and circling round them, helps throw them off balance and therefore makes it harder for them to counter-strike. Switching the clinching arm, pulling the opponent to the other side, and punching with the other arm can also be very effective.

Other clinches, takedowns and knee strikes naturally follow on from, or combine with, the dirty boxing clinch, making it very versatile. Randy Couture mastered these strategies and became one of the most successful UFC fighters.

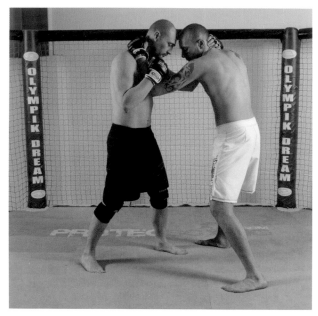

Fig 7.41 The dirty boxing clinch being applied by both competitors.

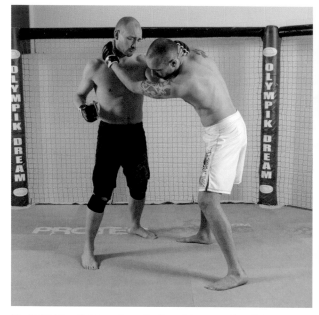

Fig 7.42 The fighter steps to the side, out of striking range, and pulls the opponent's head down.

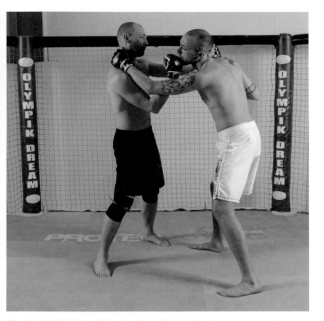

Fig 7.43 With the dirty boxing clinch in place, uppercuts can be applied. However, it is important to keep them short by using movement from the hip and leg.

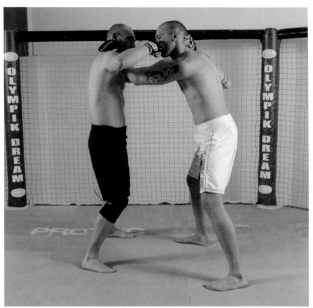

Fig 7.44 A hook to the face or body can also be applied.

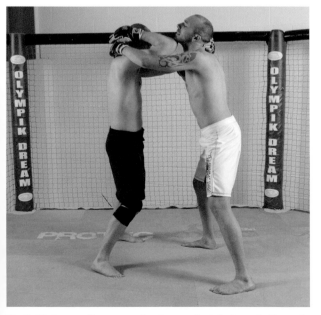

Fig 7.45 An up elbow can also be applied, but again it needs to be kept short by using movement from the hip and leg.

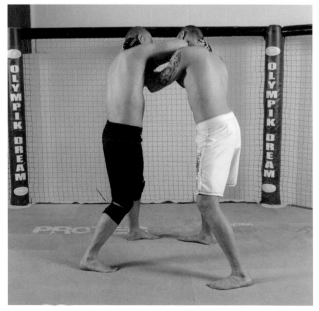

Fig 7.46 A normal elbow.

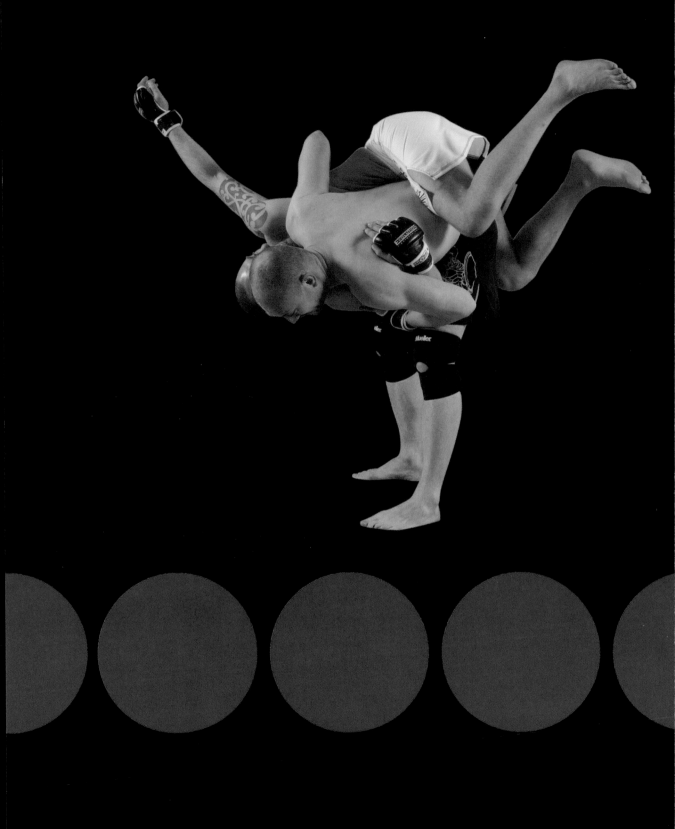

CHAPTER **EIGHT**
Takedowns

A takedown can only be attempted when an appropriate opening occurs. When it does, the fighter becomes vulnerable for a split second. To cover this vulnerability, and also to feint from the takedown to confuse the opponent, it is important to merge striking and grappling techniques.

Sweeps

Sweeps are very effective from a standing position when the opponent has all their weight on one leg, for example when kicking. However, sweeps should always be directed at the leg with the most weight on it.

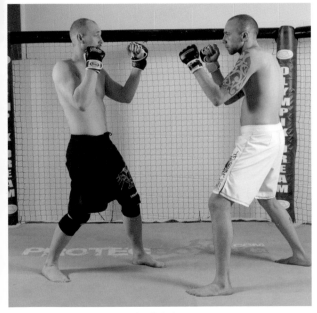

Fig 8.1 Both competitors in fighting stance.

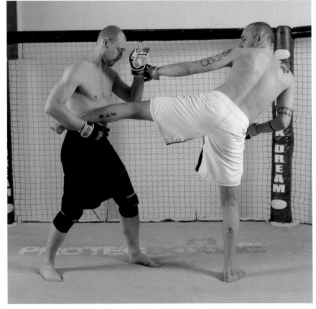

Fig 8.2 The opponent throws a roundhouse kick to the fighter's short rib. The fighter reads this and counteracts by trying to catch the kick.

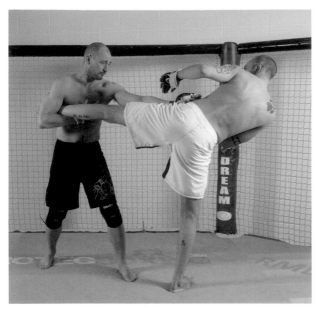

Fig 8.3 The fighter catches their opponent's leg, wrapping their arm around it and pushing them off balance with their other hand.

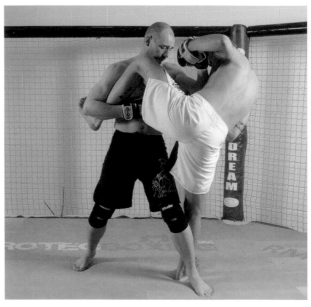

Fig 8.4 The fighter steps toward their opponent while still holding their leg and pushing them with their other hand.

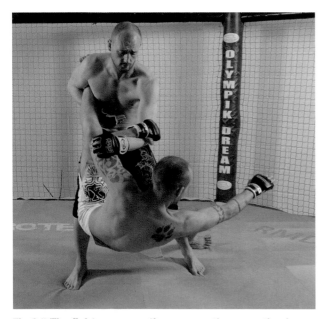

Fig 8.5 The fighter sweeps the opponent's supporting leg.

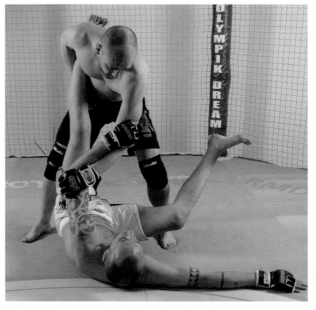

Fig 8.6 The opponent lands on their back.

Throws

Throws are integral to MMA and are used in a variety of ways. Simplicity is the key as the opponent may strike, clinch or perform a takedown at any time.

UNDER HOOK THROW

With this throw the fighter applies an under hook with one hand and holds the opponent's wrist with the other. The fighter then steps in close with their back and both heels turned toward the opponent. Forward movement of the opponent's body is then created by pulling on their wrist and maintaining the under hook. The fighter also kicks backwards with their leg just below the hip of the opponent, who then falls over it.

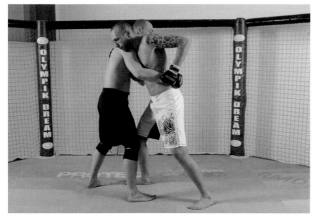

Fig 8.7 The fighter applies the one-arm under hook and wrist hold.

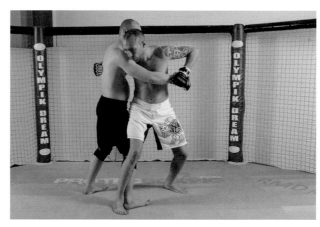

Fig 8.8 The fighter turns their back and both heels toward the opponent to make the throw easier.

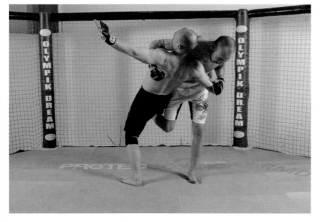

Fig 8.9 The fighter's kicked-back leg provides the pivot for the opponent to fall forward, while the under hook and wrist hold provide the force.

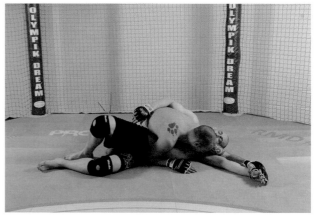

Fig 8.10 The throw can be followed by other moves including the side mount position.

UPPER BODY THROW

The throw starts in a neutral position with one arm in the under hook and the other over the opponent's arm. The opponent could also be in the same position. The leg of the fighter, on the side the throw will be executed, steps past the opponent's feet. The fighter's body is turned at the same time and the opponent is thrown over the fighter's hip.

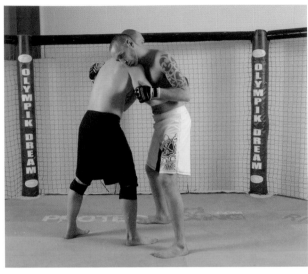

Fig 8.11 Both competitors in a single under hook where neither has the advantage.

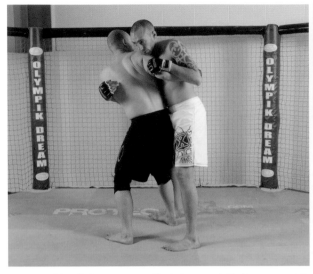

Fig 8.12 The fighter moves their leg past their opponent's feet turning their hips.

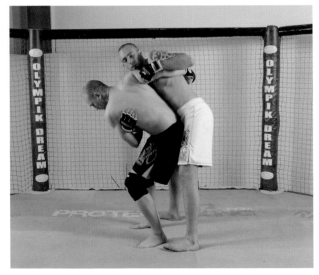

Fig 8.13 The fighter is fully turned, with both feet fairly close together and the knees bent in preparation to lift and pivot the opponent over the hip.

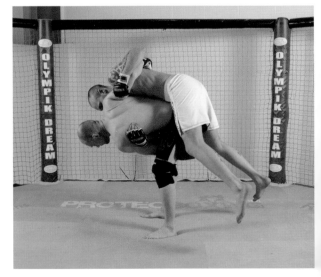

Fig 8.14 The opponent is lifted on to the fighter's hip by the fighter straightening their legs, pulling the opponent over their hip and twisting.

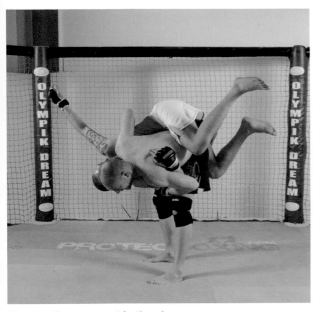

Fig 8.15 The opponent in the air.

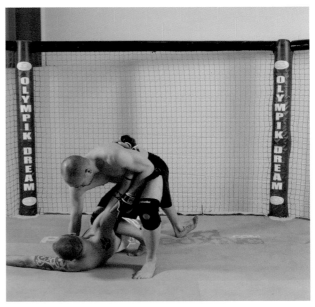

Fig 8.16 The opponent is thrown to the floor.

Leg takedowns

For the single or double-leg takedown to be effective, it is important to be within arm's length of the opponent and with a correct set-up. The success rate also increases when the move is combined with strikes. When going in for the move, the hands remain up until the head has made contact with the opponent's body. With the hands high, the fighter is less vulnerable to strikes, kicks and knees. This is particularly important when the fighter's body is moving forward as this increases the impact of blows received.

SINGLE-LEG TAKEDOWN

A single-leg takedown is normally executed when the opponent has one leg forward and the other back. In this situation a double-leg takedown would be inappropriate: the fighter would become vulnerable when travelling the further distance required to capture both legs, during which time the opponent would react and counter.

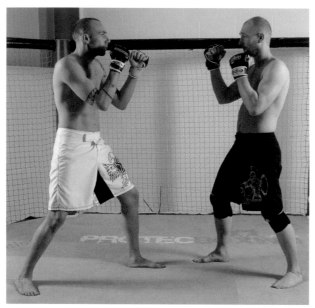

Fig 8.17 The opponent in the normal stance, one leg in front and one behind. When the opponent's legs 'mirror' those of the fighter, as above, the ideal opportunity for a single-leg take down is created.

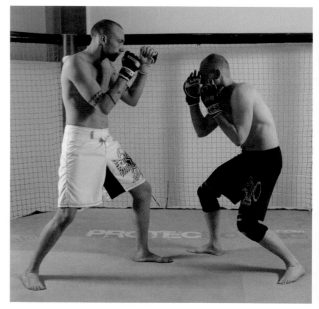

Fig 8.18 The fighter drops their body and steps to the outside of the opponent's lead foot.

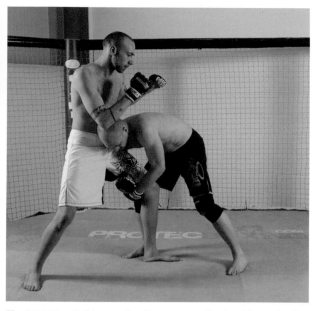

Fig 8.19 The fighter grabs the opponent's front leg, placing their head in the centre of the opponent's chest and pushing off their back leg.

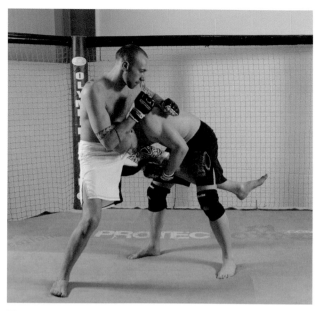

Fig 8.20 The fighter pulls the opponent's leg to their chest and brings their elbows together. The fighter's legs are now bent.

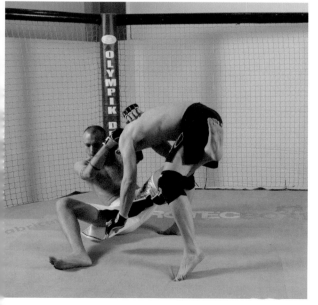

Fig 8.21 The fighter's head continues to push into the opponent's chest as they rotate their body, and the opponent falls backwards over the fighter's leg.

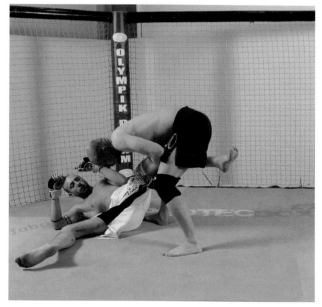

Fig 8.22 The fighter continues to push their head into the opponent's body and rotates them to the floor.

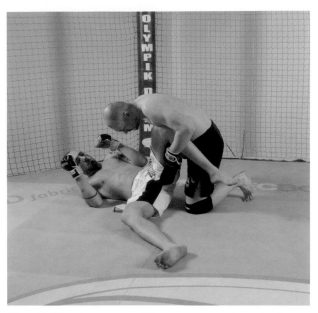 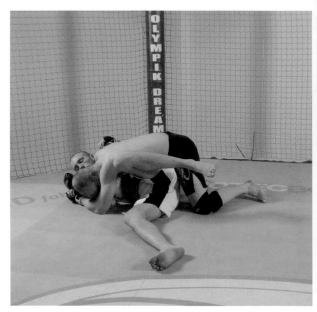

Fig 8.23 When both competitors are on the floor, the fighter tries to get on to their knees.

Fig 8.24 Once the fighter is on their knees, they secure the situation by using the top position.

DOUBLE-LEG TAKEDOWN

A double-leg takedown is normally executed when both competitors have the same stance and therefore the same lead leg. When going in for the shoot, it is important to keep the forward momentum while securing both legs with the arms. If possible, the opponent should be pushed sideways to keep away from counter-strikes, known as *guards*. Once on the ground, the opponent should be secured by using the side control position.

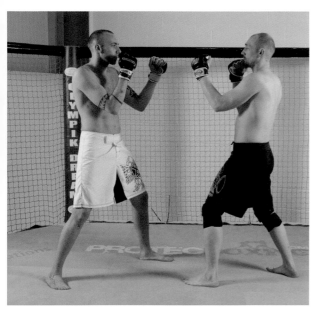

Fig 8.25 Both competitors lead with the same leg in the normal fighting stance.

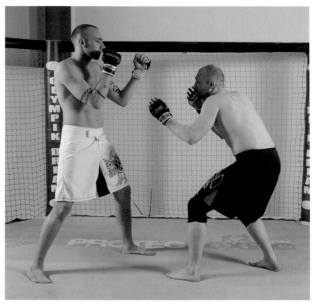

Fig 8.26 The fighter moves into a crouched stance.

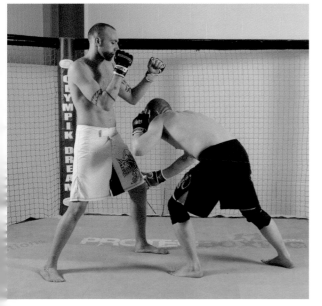

Fig 8.27 Pushing off with their back leg, the fighter explodes forward while keeping their hands up to protect against strikes. The front leg steps forward and is placed between the opponent's legs.

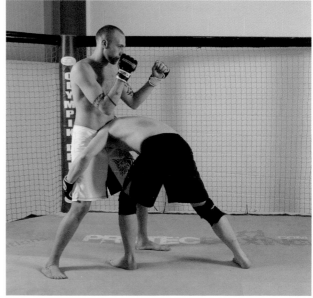

Fig 8.28 The fighter's head is placed on the side of the opponent's body, on the same side as their leading leg. Both arms are wrapped around the back of the opponent's knees.

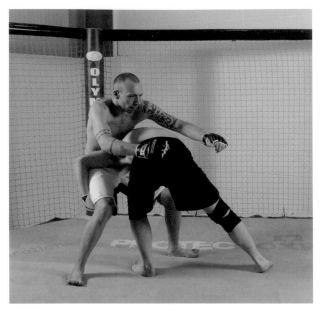

Fig 8.29 The fighter drives forward by stepping toward the opponent with their back leg. The fighter's torso is fairly straight and the shoulder and front knee are vertically aligned.

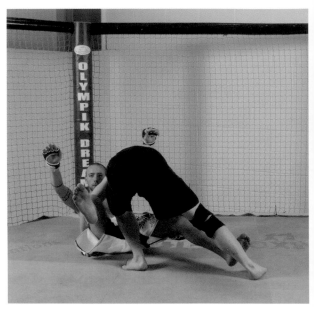

Fig 8.30 All of the fighter's weight is pushed sideways into the body of the opponent, whose leading leg is pulled into the fighter's body.

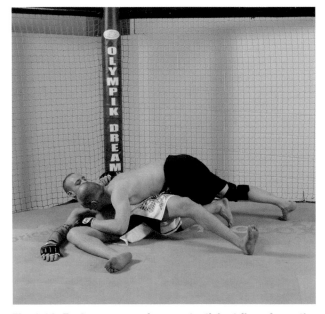

Fig 8.31 To keep away from potential strikes from the opponent's guard, the fighter stays to the side.

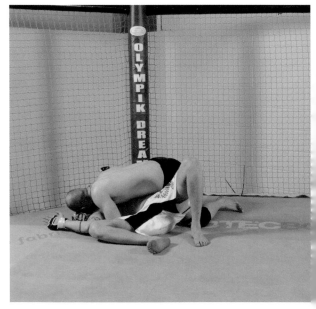

Fig 8.32 The fighter establishes the side control position.

Body lock takedown

A body lock takedown follows a successful double under hook where a tight grip around the opponent's body has been achieved. This is a very effective takedown that can seriously injure the opponent when they land.

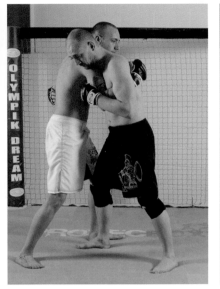

Fig 8.33 Both competitors try to establish a double under hook.

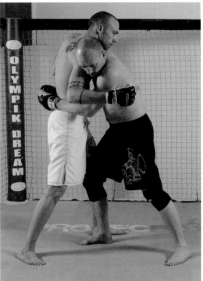

Fig 8.34 The fighter achieves the double under hook with a firm grip of their wrist.

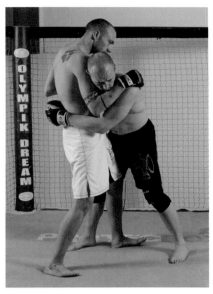

Fig 8.35 The fighter steps behind the opponent with their back leg.

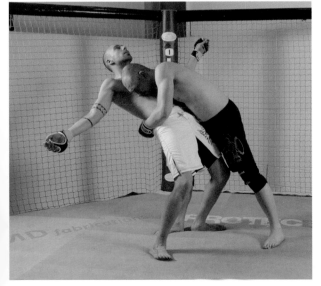

Fig 8.36 The opponent is rotated and tripped backwards by the fighter, who maintains a strong grip.

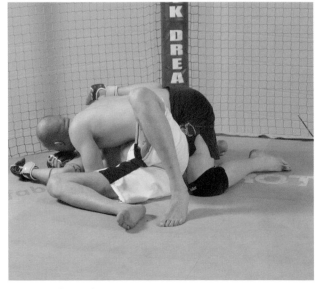

Fig 8.37 Once the opponent is on their back, the fighter secures the side control position.

Takedown from the Muay Thai clinch

If the fighter has been unable to bring their opponent's head down to apply strikes, they can use their resistance against them by releasing their grip and shooting in for a takedown.

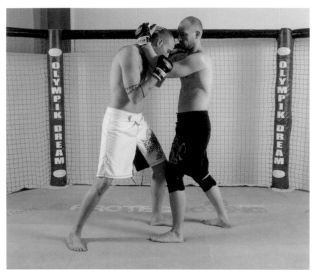

Fig 8.38 The fighter holds their opponent in a Muay Thai clinch.

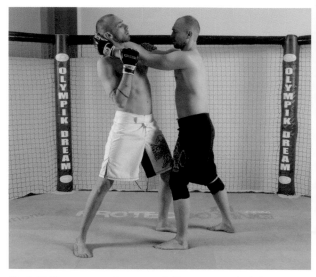

Fig 8.39 The opponent successfully prevents their head from being pulled forward, so the fighter releases their hold.

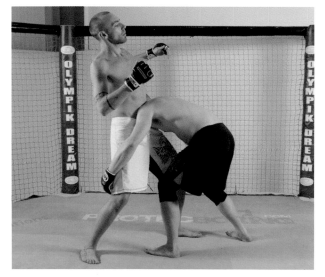

Fig 8.40 Released from the hold, the opponent's body moves backwards and the fighter shoots in for a double-leg takedown.

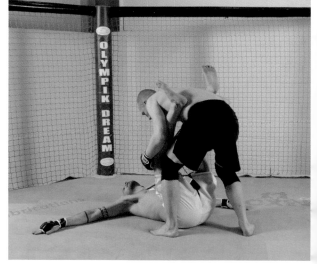

Fig 8.41 The opponent is slammed to the ground.

Body lock takedown from the back

An opponent held from the back in a body lock becomes very vulnerable to a takedown. This is a simple manoeuvre for the fighter, involving wrapping their leg around their opponent's and applying their body weight until they collapse to the ground. Once on the ground, the fighter can apply a rear naked choke.

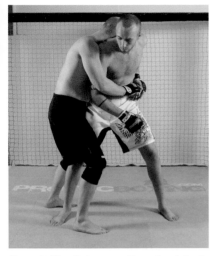

Fig 8.42 The fighter applies a back body lock with one arm of the opponent secured.

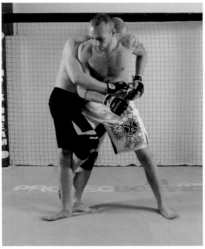

Fig 8.43 On the same side as the secured arm, the fighter wraps their leg around their opponent's.

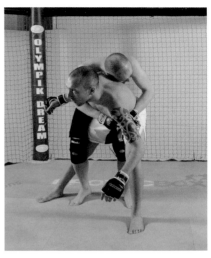

Fig 8.44 Keeping in close contact with the opponent, the fighter applies their weight while pushing forward, thereby forcing the opponent to the ground.

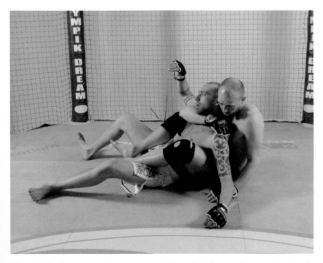

Fig 8.45 Once on the ground, the fighter rolls on to their back, taking their opponent with them and securing their legs by hooking them with their own.

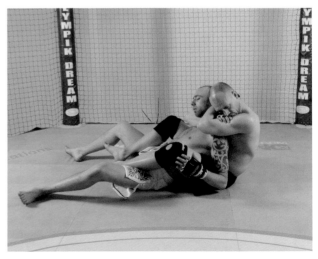

Fig 8.46 The fighter applies a rear naked choke hold.

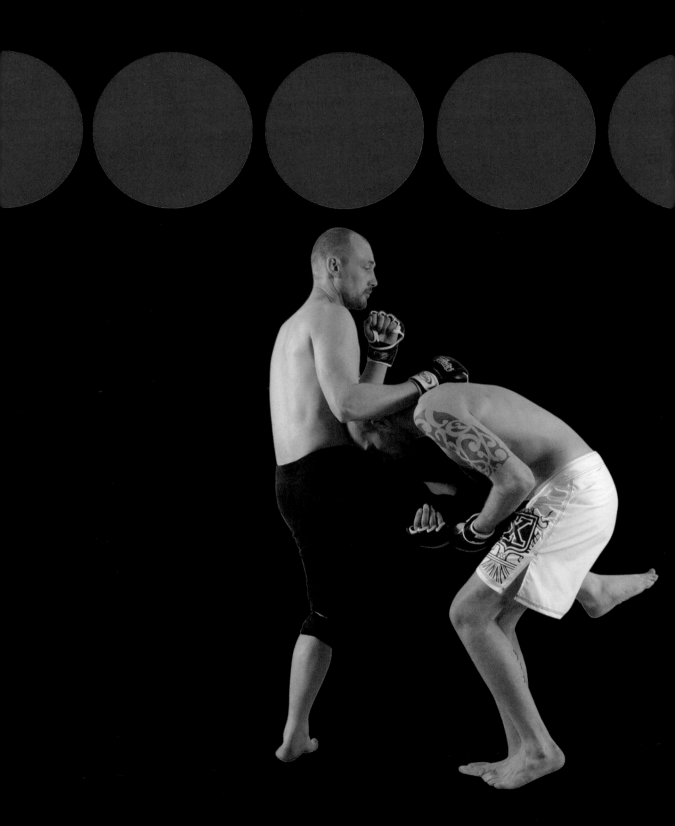

CHAPTER **NINE**
Defence against takedowns

A good defence against takedowns is essential for fighters who are more vulnerable on the ground, for example grapplers and strikers.

Takedown defence principle

The basic defence principle is the same for all takedowns: step aside and avoid contact by deflecting the opponent with a push. This also puts them off balance and provides the opportunity to apply a punch, strike or takedown.

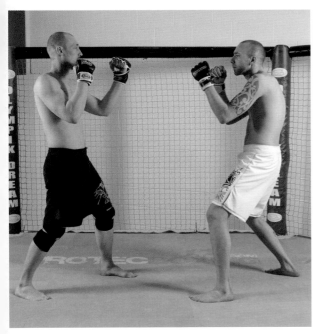

Fig 9.1 The competitors in fighting stance.

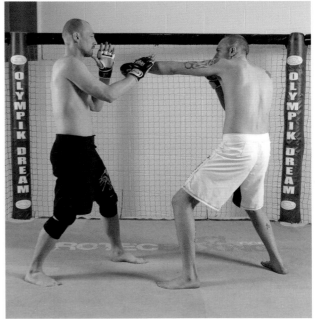

Fig 9.2 The opponent attempts a jab to distract the fighter, who parries.

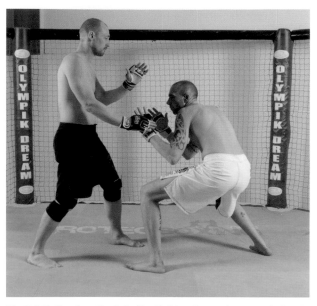

Fig 9.3 Following the jab, the fighter drops down and shoots in for a takedown.

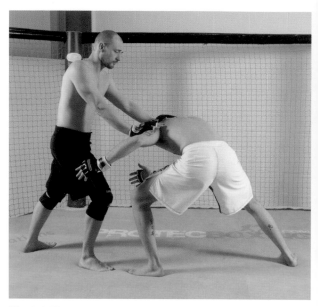

Fig 9.4 The opponent responds by placing their forearm around the fighter's neck and moving their legs out of the fighter's reach. The fighter steps backwards and the opponent's momentum takes them forward into the space created.

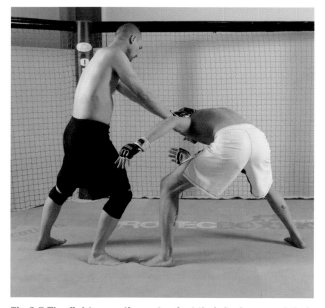

Fig 9.5 The fighter continues to pivot their body around their opponent's to keep out of their reach.

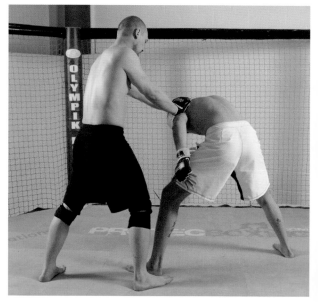

Fig 9.6 While pivoting, the fighter is pushing their opponent off base, creating the perfect moment for a strike or takedown.

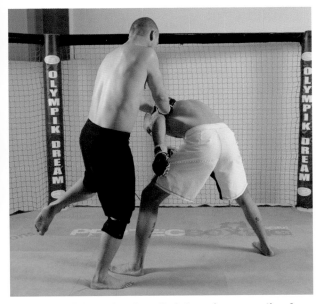

Fig 9.7 The fighter chambers their knee in preparation for a strike.

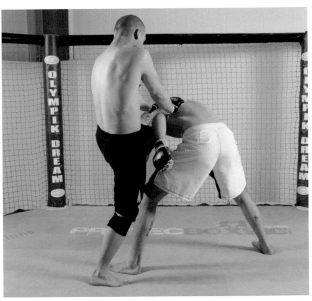

Fig 9.8 The fighter strikes a devastating knee to the head.

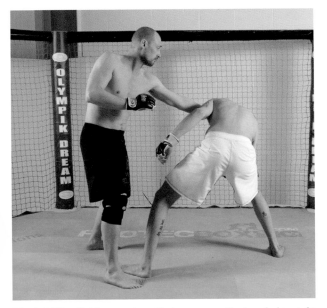

Fig 9.9 The fighter pushes their opponent's head down in preparation for a cross to the head.

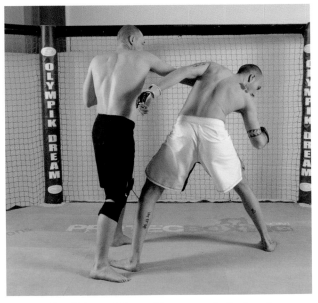

Fig 9.10 The fighter strikes with a cross to the head.

Guillotine choke to defend against a leg takedown

The guillotine choke can be used by the fighter as a defence move if their opponent is shooting in for a takedown. As the opponent comes in, it is too late to defend against them with other techniques, but because the opponent is likely to have their head down, it provides a good position for the guillotine choke to be applied.

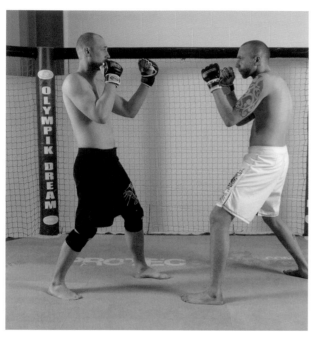

Fig 9.11 Both competitors are in the fighting stance.

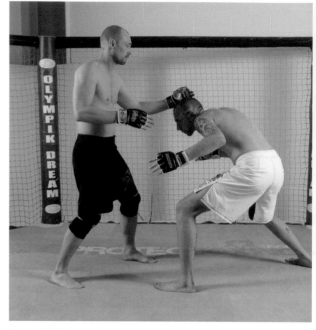

Fig 9.12 The opponent shoots in for a double-leg takedown. As the opponent's hands are low their neck is exposed, providing a good opportunity for the fighter to apply the guillotine choke.

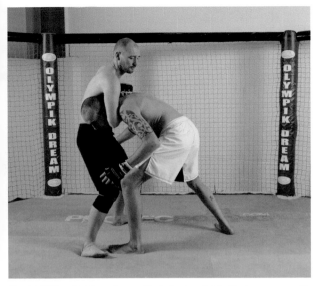

Fig 9.13 The fighter places their feet outside their opponent's and wraps their arm around the opponent's neck.

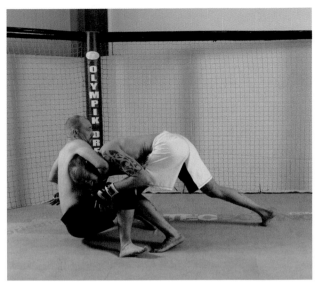

Fig 9.14 The opponent drives the fighter to the ground. The fighter attempts to keep their legs away from their opponent's body so that they can later be wrapped around them.

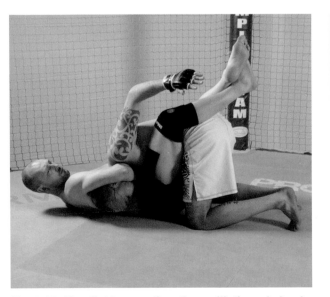

Fig 9.15 The fighter applies the guillotine choke by tightening their arms around the neck. The legs are wrapped around the opponent's body and interlocked. By pushing the opponent away with the legs and applying the choke, the opponent is likely to be forced to tap out.

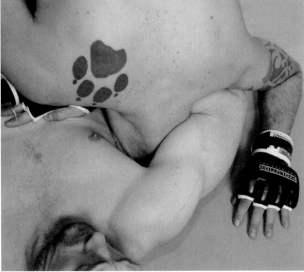

Fig 9.16 The correct neck position.

The sprawl

The sprawl can be used as a last resort when an opponent penetrates too far with a takedown. To prevent the opponent grasping the back of the fighter's legs, they step and push back with their legs until their legs and hips are flat to the ground. The feet are also flattened to help keep the hips down and to prevent the body from involuntarily rising if pushed. This can also help trap the opponent under their weight. From this position the fighter can slide backwards, again to prevent the opponent reaching their legs.

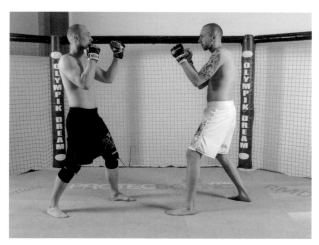

Fig 9.17 Both competitors are in the fighting stance.

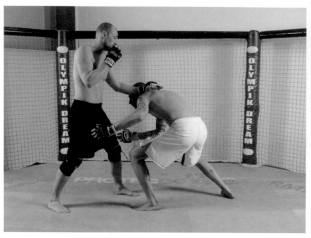

Fig 9.18 The opponent shoots forward for a double-leg takedown. The fighter reacts by lowering to a crouched stance.

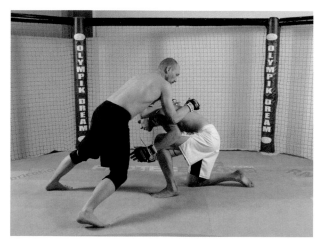

Fig 9.19 The fighter's elbow is bent on their leading side and catches the opponent's shoulder in the crook. The leg on the same side as the crooked arm is pushed backwards so all their weight is on the opponent.

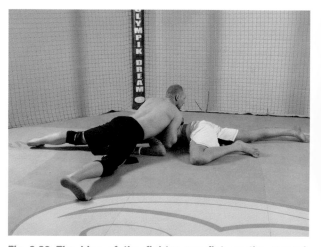

Fig 9.20 The hips of the fighter are flat on the ground, preventing the opponent from grabbing them.

Defence against a single-leg takedown

Balance is very important when defending against a single-leg takedown as techniques are applied while being pushed about on one leg. In this technique the opponent's head is pushed away to the side, and then down from the fighter's body in order to roll them to the ground.

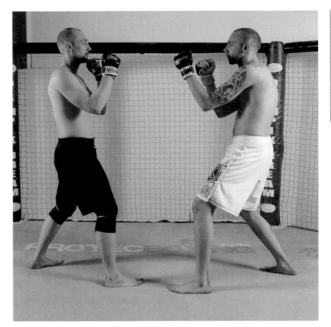

Fig 9.21 Both competitors are in the fighting stance.

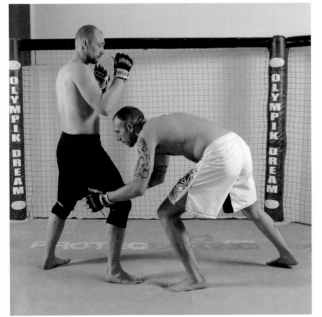

Fig 9.22 The opponent goes in for a single-leg takedown.

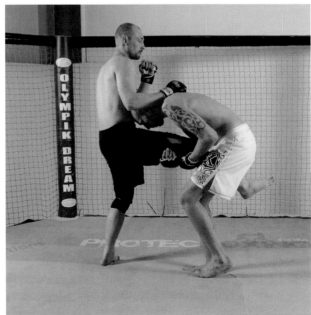

Fig 9.23 The opponent holds on to the lead leg.

93

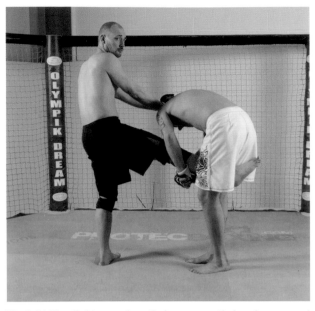

Fig 9.24 The fighter pushes their opponent's head away and to the side with their hands.

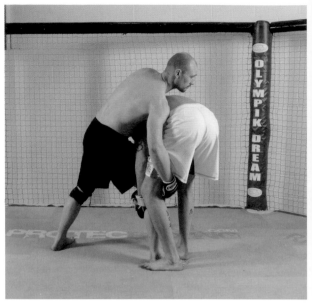

Fig 9.25 The opponent's head is pushed from the fighter's side towards the ground while the fighter's other arm wraps around the opponent's leg.

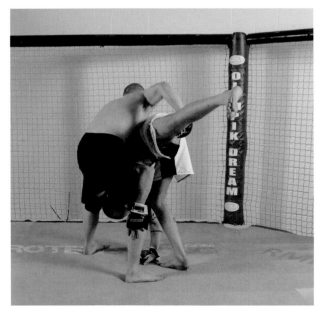

Fig 9.26 The opponent's head is pushed down and their leg pulled upward, forcing them into a forward roll.

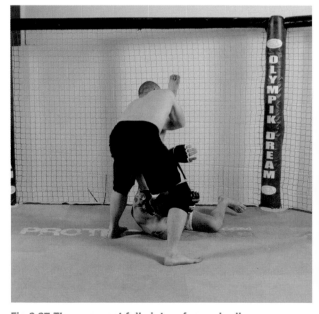

Fig 9.27 The opponent falls into a forward roll.

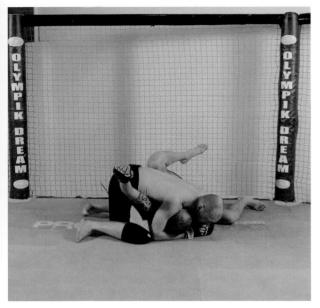

Fig 9.28 The opponent is followed to the ground and held in the side control position.

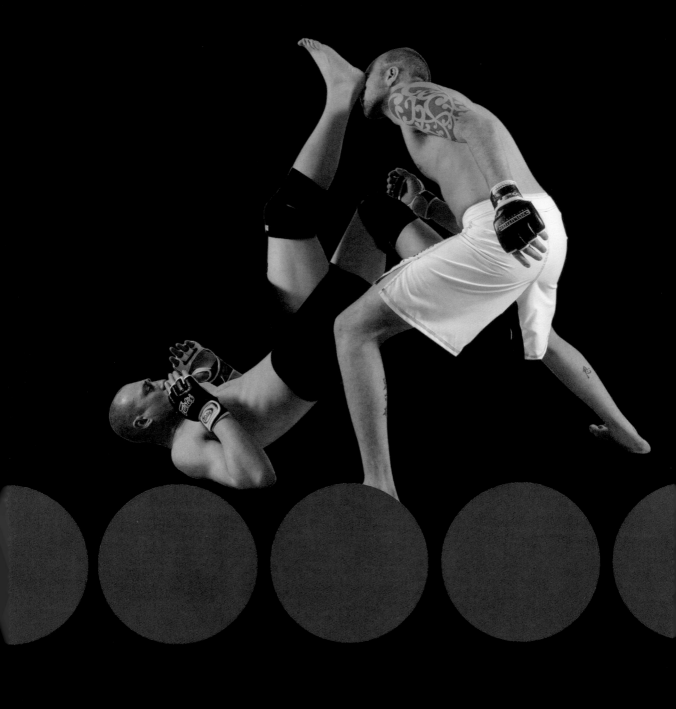

CHAPTER **TEN**
Fighting from the ground

Fighters are very vulnerable when they are on the ground and their opponent is still standing. They must therefore get back on to their feet as quickly as possible, but also ensure that when on the ground their opponent does not take control of their legs.

Shell

The shell position is created by lying on the back and bringing the elbows and knees together and the hands up to the face. This creates a line of defence down both sides of the body and helps protect against strikes or kicks to the body or face. From this position it is also possible to apply upward kicks, ideally with the sole of the foot directly toward the opponent.

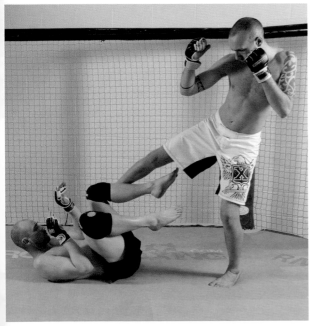

Fig 10.1 The fighter in the shell position defending and blocking kicks mainly with the shin.

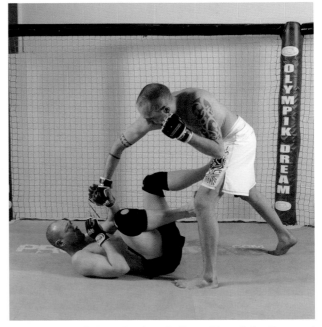

Fig 10.2 The fighter in the shell position defending and blocking punches with their hands.

Kicking while in the shell

Although the shell is a defensive position, it is still possible for an attacking kick to be applied.

STOMP KICK TO THE UPPER KNEE

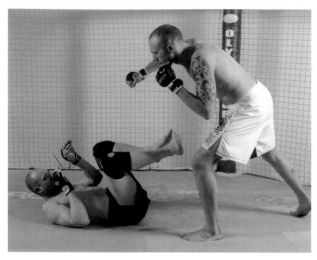

Fig 10.3 The fighter is attacked in the shell position.

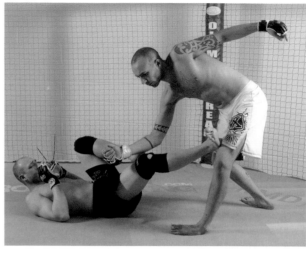

Fig 10.4 The fighter counter-attacks with a stomp kick to just above the opponent's knee to hyperextend it.

KICK TO THE HEAD

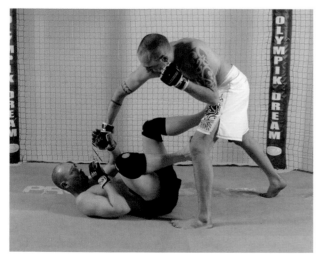

Fig 10.5 The opponent closes the gap with the fighter on the ground. The fighter waits for the opponent's head to come closer and prepares for the move by placing their elbows on the ground.

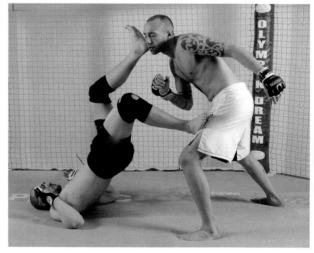

Fig 10.6 The fighter uses their elbows to push off the ground while thrusting their leg upward to make contact with their opponent's head with their heel. This move can result in a knockout.

HEEL KICK

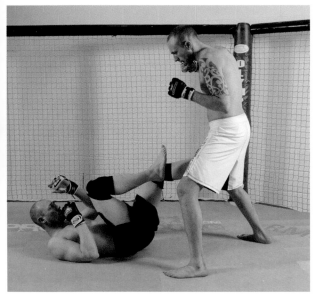

Fig 10.7 While on the floor, the fighter places one leg on the opponent's thigh.

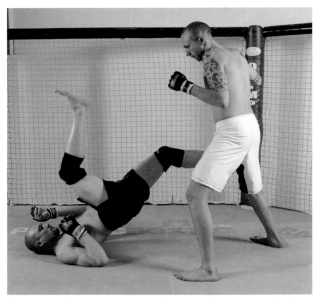

Fig 10.8 The fighter raises their hips off the ground by pushing on this leg and rolling back on to their shoulders.

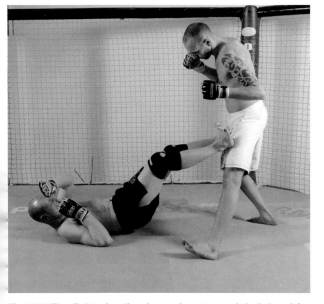

Fig 10.9 The fighter's other leg swings toward their head for extra momentum, then comes down to place a strike with the heel on the opponent's thigh.

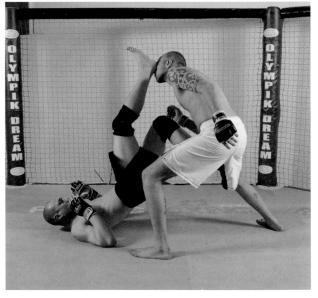

Fig 10.10 If the opponent's head is low enough the kick can also be applied there.

PUSH KICK

This is a good technique to use if the opponent has gained control of the feet, which is a very vulnerable position for the fighter to be in.

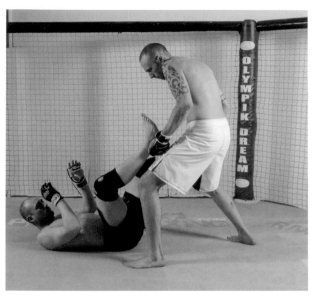

Fig 10.11 The opponent controls both of the fighter's legs.

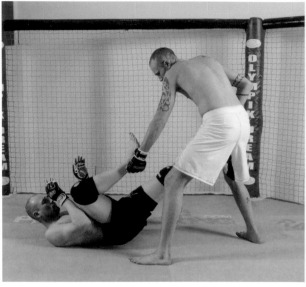

Fig 10.12 The fighter pushes one leg toward the opponent's body to loosen their grip.

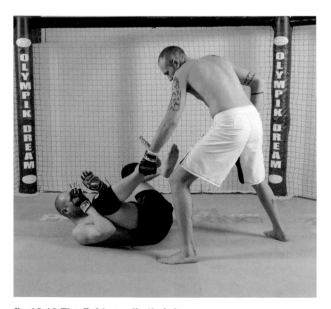

fig 10.13 The fighter pulls their leg away.

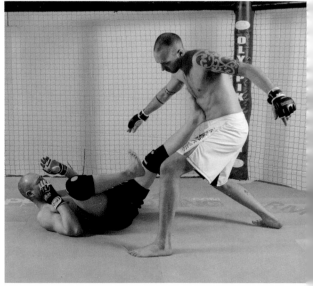

Fig 10.14 The fighter thrusts their leg into the midsection of their opponent using a push kick.

De La Riva

Another option to use when on the ground is the De La Riva. This involves wrapping one leg around the opponent's lead leg and pressing the foot of the other leg into their midsection. Further stability is gained by gripping the heel of the opponent's lead foot with the hand. The benefits for the fighter are increased control over their opponent and management of distance between them.

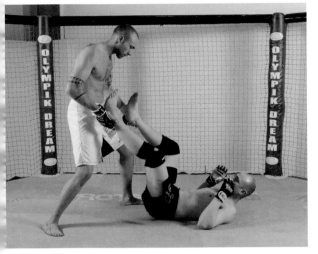

Fig 10.15 The opponent has the advantage because they are controlling the fighter's legs.

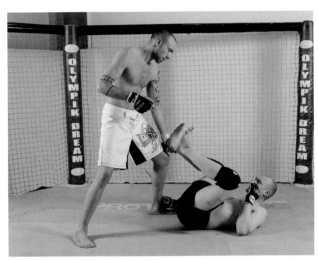

Fig 10.16 The fighter escapes the grip.

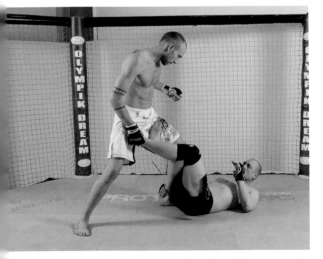

Fig 10.17 The fighter presses one foot into the opponent's midsection while the other leg wraps around the outside of their lead leg, and the fighter's right hand is placed on the opponent's lead leg.

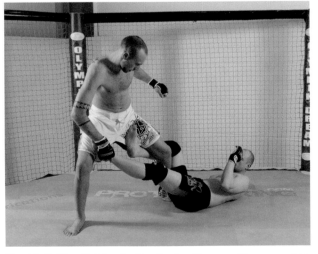

Fig 10.18 The fighter in the De La Riva position now has more control over the opponent.

Kicking while in the De La Riva

If when in the De La Riva position the opponent tries to attack with a punch, the foot placed in the midsection can be used to keep them away or to place a kick.

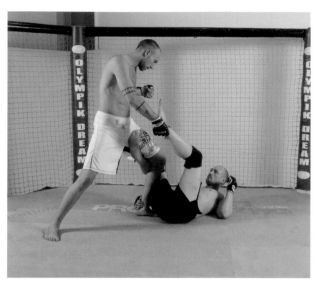

Fig 10.19 The opponent is secured in the De La Riva position.

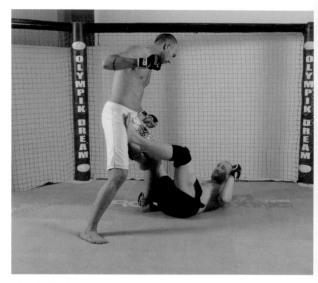

Fig 10.20 The opponent attempts an overhand throw.

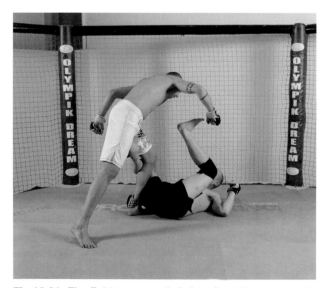

Fig 10.21 The fighter moves their foot from the opponent's midsection and chambers their leg.

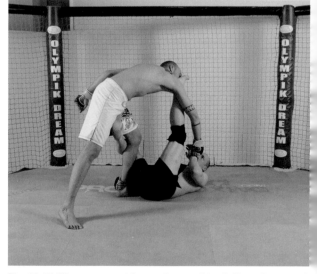

Fig 10.22 The opponent leans forward to deliver the punch as the fighter counter-attacks with a kick to their face. During the move the fighter maintains the guard to their face in case the punch makes it through.

De La Riva sweep

If the captured opponent moves forward to throw an overhand, the fighter can curl up into a half shell to protect themselves from the blow and use the momentum of the opponent to bring them to the ground. The fighter also takes control of the opponent's head to maximise the effect.

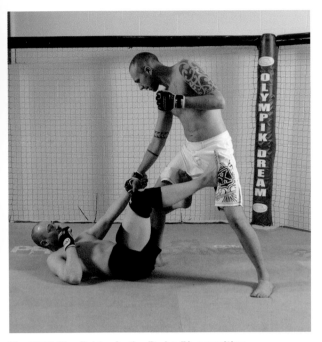

Fig 10.23 The fighter in the De La Riva position.

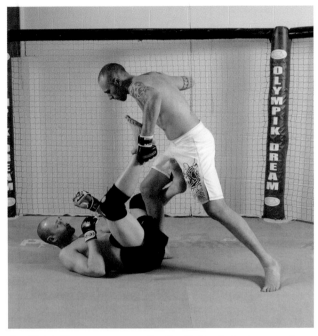

Fig 10.24 The opponent pulls the fighter's foot away from their midsection. The opponent's other hand is preparing for an overhand throw.

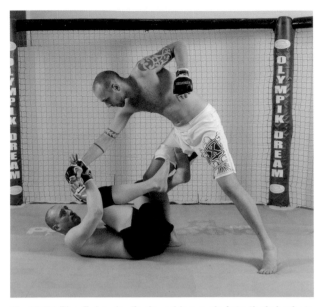

Fig 10.25 The fighter's displaced leg curls into their body to protect against the attack. The elbow on the same side is brought to the knee to form the half shell, but with the hand raised to catch the strike.

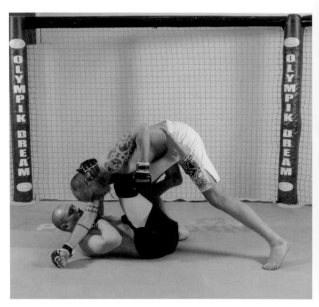

Fig 10.26 The opponent's overhand passes the fighter and their momentum brings them down. The fighter grabs the back of the opponent's head and keeps their leg wrapped around the opponent's.

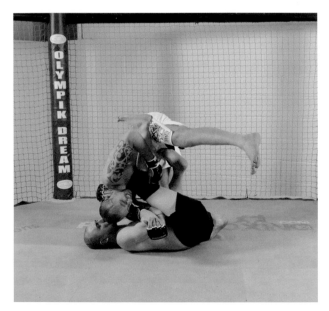

Fig 10.27 The leg wrapped around the opponent's is used to pull them toward the ground, while the foot of the other leg is placed on their hip.

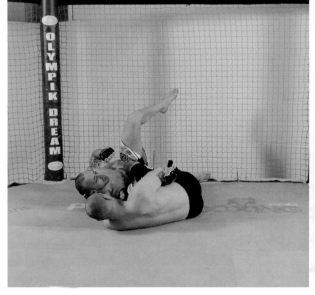

Fig 10.28 The opponent's body is pushed over and to the side of the fighter's.

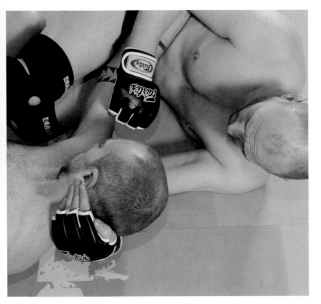

Fig 10.29 The grip on the opponent's head is maintained throughout.

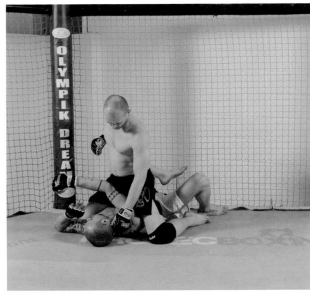

Fig 10.30 The fighter uses this grip to pull themselves up on to their knees.

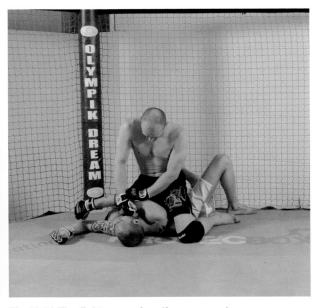

Fig 10.31 The fighter punches the opponent.

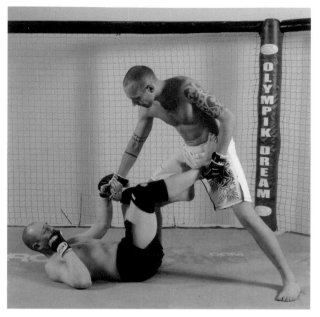

Fig 10.32 The fighter in the De La Riva position.

De La Riva to closed guard

The fighter performing a De La Riva can initially protect themselves from an overhand throw by curling up into the shell. The fighter can then counter-attack by controlling the opponent's head and either applying a sweep if there is enough momentum, or a full guard.

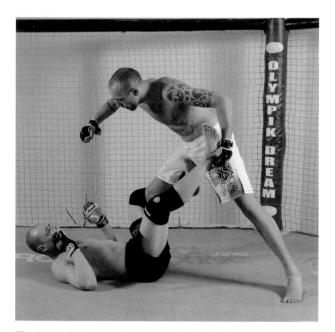

Fig 10.33 The opponent pulls the fighter's foot away from their midsection with one hand and throws an overhand with the other.

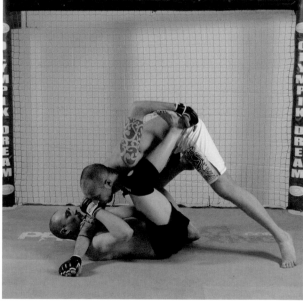

Fig 10.34 The fighter's displaced leg curls into their body to protect against the attack. The elbow on the same side is brought to the knee to form the half shell, but with their hand raised to catch the strike.

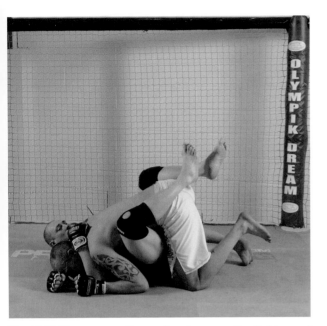

Fig 10.35 The opponent's overhand passes the fighter and their momentum brings them down. The fighter grabs the back of the opponent's head and keeps their leg wrapped around the opponent's.

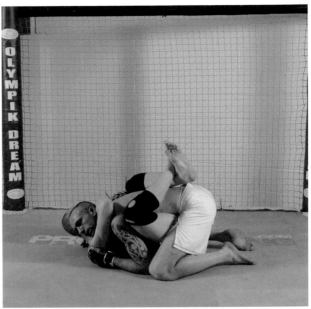

Fig 10.36 If there is not enough momentum to sweep the opponent, the fighter holds them in a closed guard where the fighter's head is controlled and the legs are gripped around their torso.

De La Riva to guard

Transition between the De La Riva and the goes guard is straightforward. However, it should only be held for a short period as it is relatively easy to defend against by the opponent either whipping away the foot placed on their hip or stepping backwards with the back leg. When used correctly, it is an important lead into sweeping an opponent.

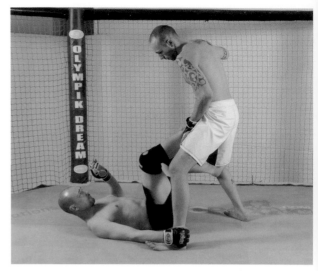

Fig 10.37 The opponent is held in the goes guard. The fighter's foot is placed on the hip of the opponent's leading leg, with the heel of the same leg being held by the fighter's hand. The fighter's other foot hooks the back of the knee of the opponent's other leg.

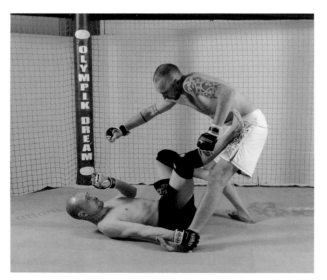

Fig 10.38 A successful sweep is accomplished by the fighter completing three simultaneous moves: pushing the opponent back with the foot placed on the hip; collapsing the knee of the opponent's back leg by pulling the knee with the foot; and pulling the opponent's heel with the hand.

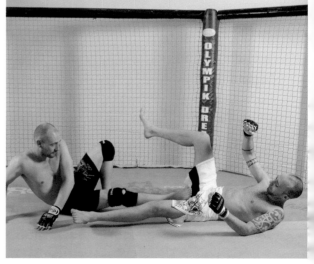

Fig 10.39 The opponent falls backwards and is forced to the ground.

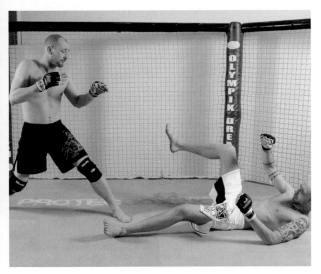

Fig 10.40 The fighter takes the opportunity to get back on to their feet.

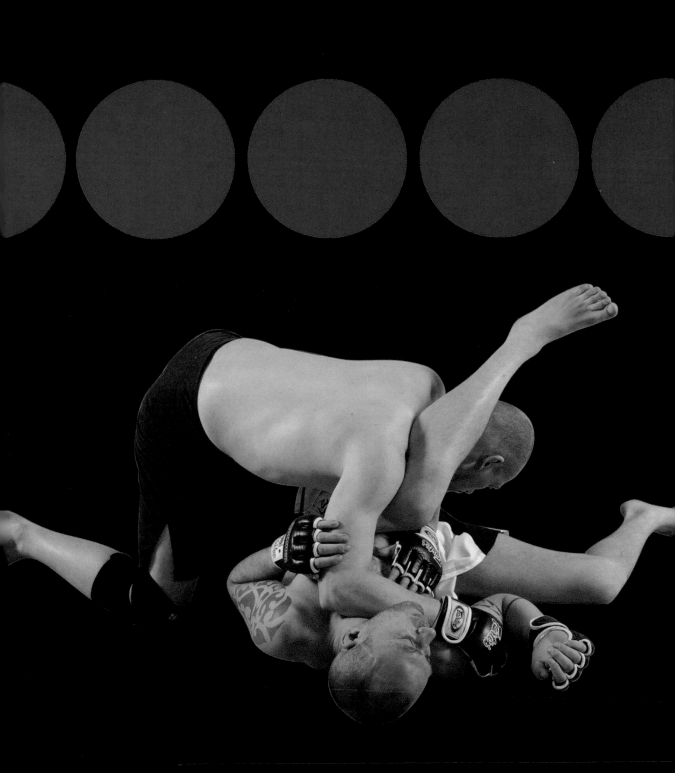

CHAPTER **ELEVEN**
Guard top

When both competitors are on the ground with the fighter on top between their opponent's legs, this is described as being in the *guard top* position. From this position, the fighter can strike with either their hands or elbows. The opponent in the *guard bottom* position will either try to sweep the fighter or control their head and hands to minimise the amount of weight they can put behind their strikes.

Posture up guard

The fighter places one hand on the opponent's chest to prevent them from sitting up and taking hold of their head. With this control in place, the fighter can apply strikes with the full power of their body weight. The fighter maintains good posture and a solid base by sitting upright.

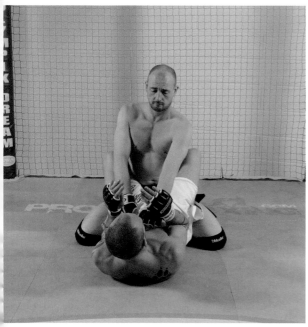

Fig 11.1 The fighter pushes the opponent's chest down with one hand while maintaining good posture.

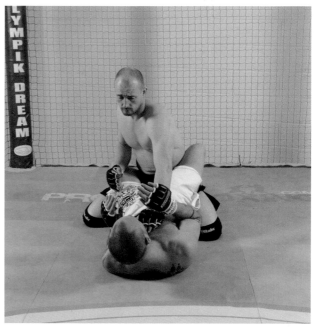

Fig 11.2 The fighter's other hand remains back to provide the option of strikes or to push the opponent's legs apart.

Bicep control

The bicep control prevents the opponent from sitting up. When applied, the fighter's arms are straight and the hands are placed on the biceps with the thumbs on top. With their arms pinned to the mat, the opponent's options for counter techniques are reduced.

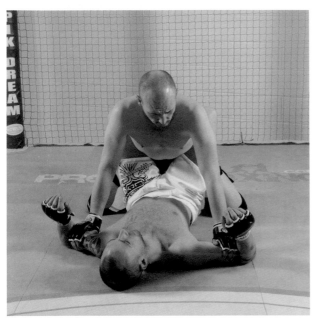 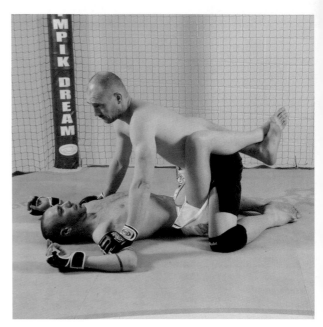

Fig 11.3 The fighter controls the biceps by pinning the opponent down with their hands, with the thumbs on top.

Fig 11.4 The fighter's arms are straight and their body is leaning forward.

Striking

The opponent on the ground aims to minimise the impact from strikes and elbows by controlling the fighter's hands and head. The fighter counteracts this by swiping away or controlling the opponent's hands. Both can use strikes to pass each other's defences.

OVERHAND

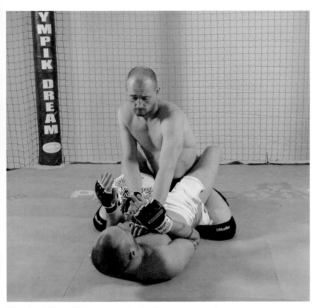

Fig 11.5 The fighter controls the opponent.

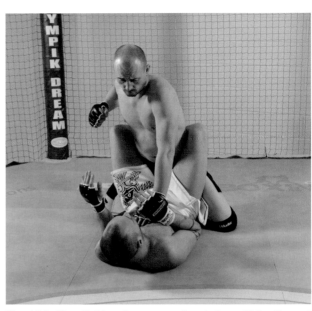

Fig 11.6 The fighter frees one hand in anticipation of punching.

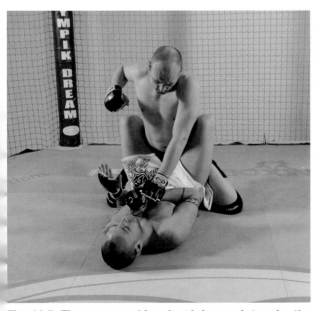

Fig 11.7 The non-punching hand is used to pin the opponent's hand to their chest, effectively preventing them from defending themselves.

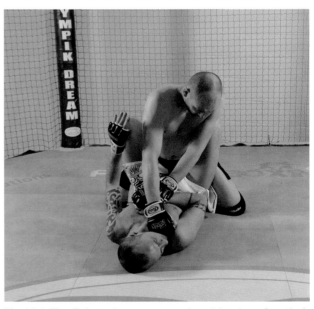

Fig 11.8 The fighter throws an overhand by dropping their weight forward.

HAMMER FIST

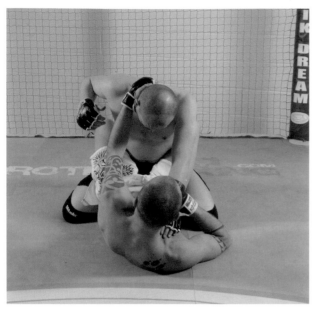

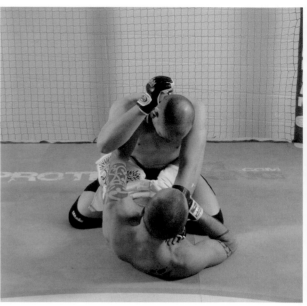

Fig 11.9 The opponent controls the fighter's head and wrist to prevent the fighter from throwing straight punches.

Fig 11.10 The side of the opponent's arm holding the fighter's head is unprotected, so the fighter pulls back their hand in preparation to throw a hammer fist.

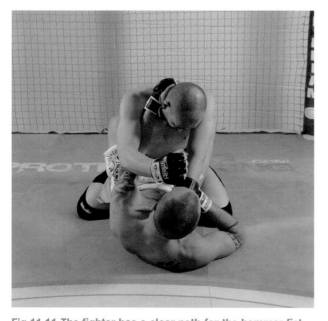

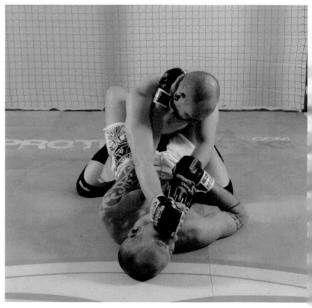

Fig 11.11 The fighter has a clear path for the hammer fist.

Fig 11.12 The hammer fist lands in the opponent's face.

UPPERCUT

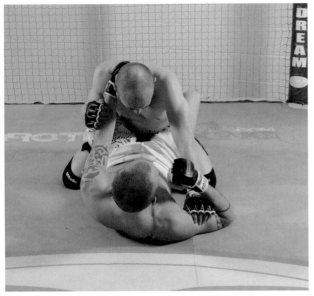

Fig 11.13 The opponent controls the fighter's head to prevent them from throwing straight punches. The fighter has one hand on the opponent's bicep to pin it to the mat.

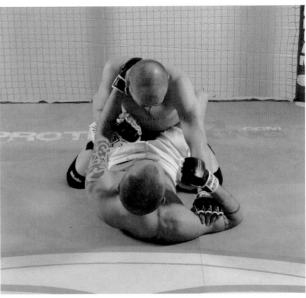

Fig 11.14 The fighter brings their other hand under the arm controlling their head.

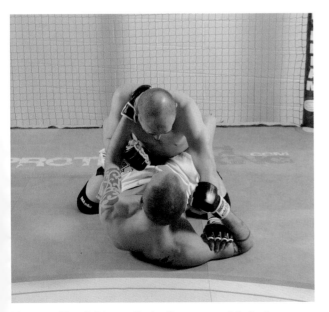

Fig 11.15 The fighter waits for the opponent to look up.

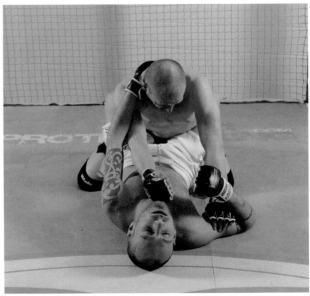

Fig 11.16 When they do, the fighter throws an uppercut to their chin.

ELBOW

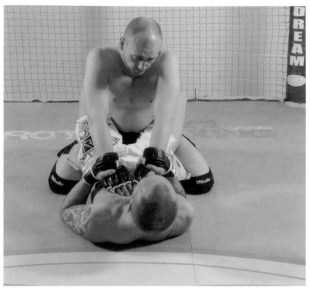

Fig 11.17 The opponent controls the fighter's hands by holding their wrists.

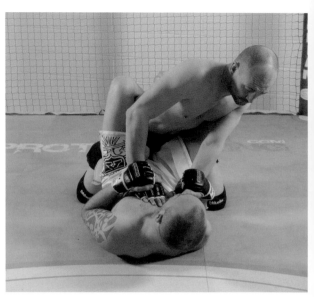

Fig 11.18 The fighter leans their body to the opposite side to the elbowing arm. The striking arm rotates upward and forward.

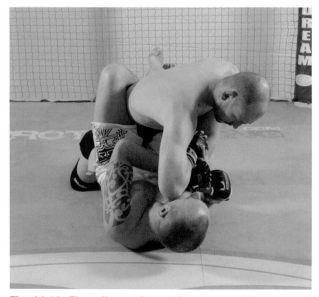

Fig 11.19 The elbow clears the opponent's arm and continues to rotate with the fighter's body weight behind it until striking the opponent in the face.

BODY-BODY-HEAD COMBINATION FROM GUARD TOP

Striking combinations in ground and pound are essential as they generate openings for strikes. The body-body-head punching combination is used to make the opponent protect the side of their body and, once they do, to punch their unprotected face. However, the non-striking arm should remain active to prevent the opponent's hips from rising or an arm bar being applied.

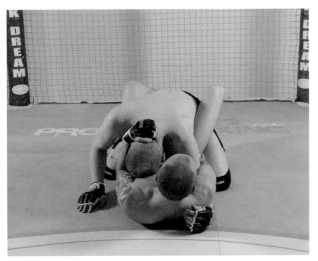

Fig 11.20 The opponent controls the fighter's head and one arm.

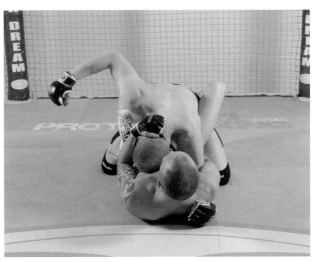

Fig 11.21 By controlling the fighter's head, the opponent leaves one side of their body exposed. The fighter plans to take advantage of this and pulls their striking arm back in preparation.

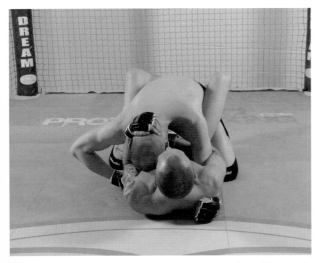

Fig 11.22 The fighter strikes the opponent's ribs with a body hook.

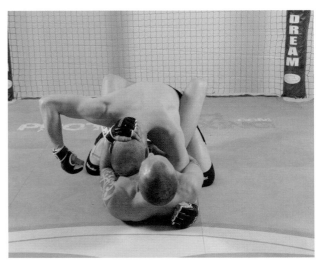

Fig 11.23 The fighter strikes again.

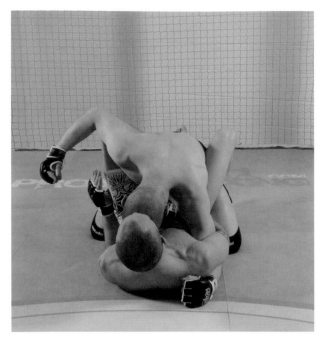

Fig 11.24 To defend against another strike, the opponent lowers their arm to protect their side.

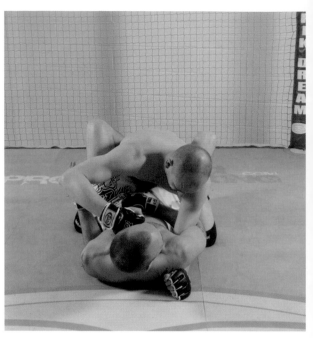

Fig 11.25 The fighter takes advantage of the space created and applies a hook to the opponent's face.

Passing the guard

The fighter is in the full guard of an opponent on the ground when the opponent has their legs locked around them. In this position the opponent has the advantage as they are able to create distance, defend against strikes and attempt submissions.

To get past this, the fighter distracts the opponent with combinations of strikes and then mixes and matches striking and specific passing-the-guard techniques.

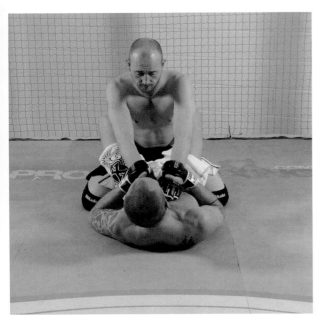

Fig 11.26 The fighter is in the opponent's full guard.

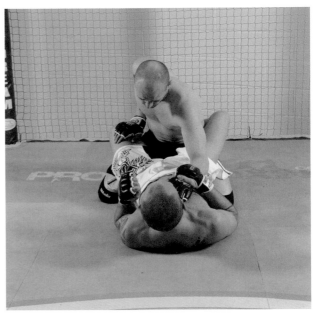

Fig 11.27 The fighter simulating a pass-the-guard attempt by pushing down on to the opponent's leg.

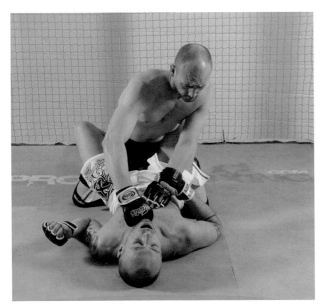

Fig 11.28 The opponent focuses their attention on their leg and the fighter uses the moment to come in with a strong overhand.

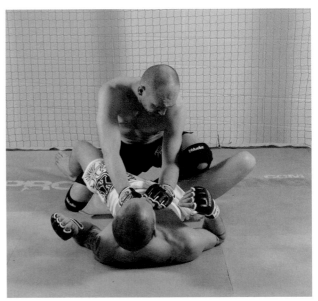

Fig 11.29 The impact of the overhand forces the opponent's leg lock to break. The fighter pushes their knee and elbow against the opponent's inner thigh to prevent the leg lock from being reapplied.

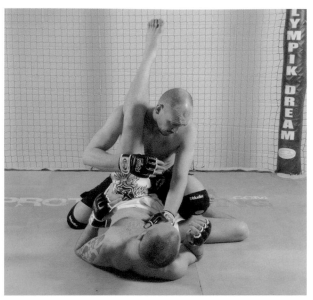

Fig 11.30 The fighter's knee and forearm push the opponent's inner thigh toward the mat. The fighter's other arm scoops to the outside of the opponent's other leg.

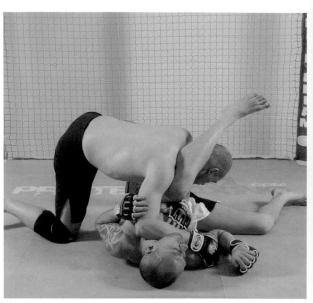

Fig 11.31 The fighter's forearm moves from the opponent's inner thigh to their shoulder, while the fighter pushes the scooped leg toward the opponent's body.

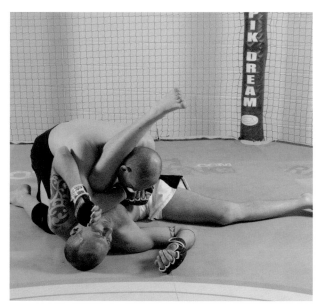

Fig 11.32 The arm with the scooped leg slides down so the opponent's leg is on the fighter's shoulder. Both hands join on the opponent's shoulder as the fighter pushes their weight forward.

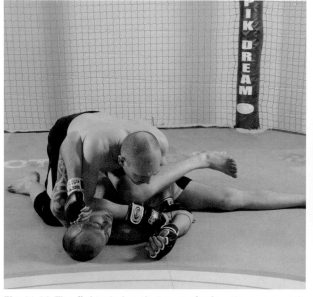

Fig 11.33 The fighter's leg that was pinning the opponent's leg to the ground now pushes the fighter's weight forward and on to the opponent's neck.

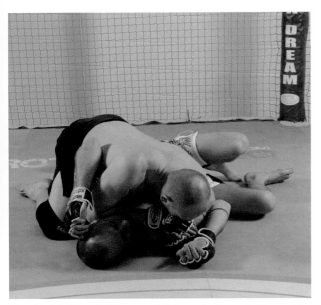

Fig 11.34 The fighter maintains their weight on the opponent's face while continuing to lower their body toward the floor.

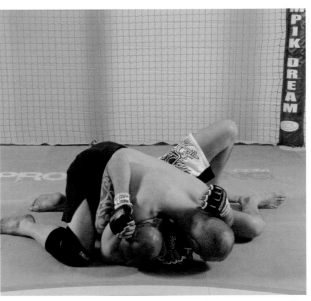

Fig 11.35 The fighter's weight is fully distributed on to the opponent's body as they assume the side control position.

Passing the guard by standing up

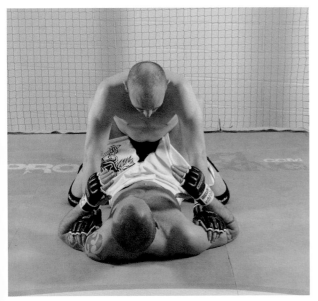

Fig 11.36 The fighter is in the opponent's full guard but controls the opponent's biceps.

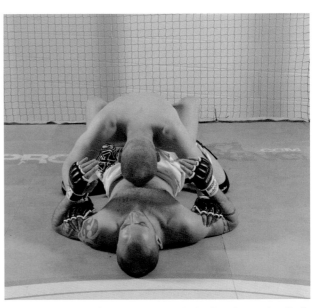

Fig 11.37 The fighter lowers their head on to their opponent's solar plexus.

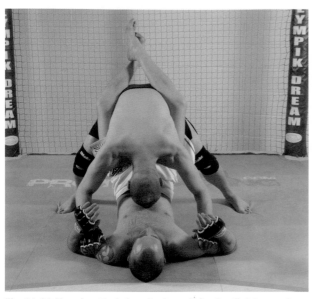

Fig 11.38 Keeping their head where it is, the fighter springs on to their feet.

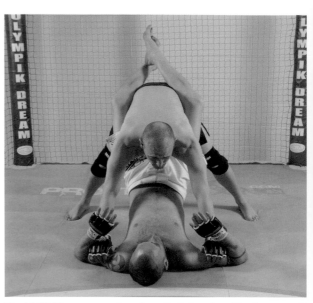

Fig 11.39 The opponent pushes their head and body upward, but the fighter's hands remain on the opponent's biceps.

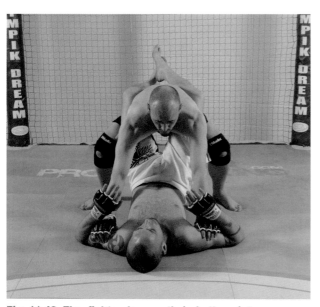

Fig 11.40 The fighter lowers their bottom into a secure stance.

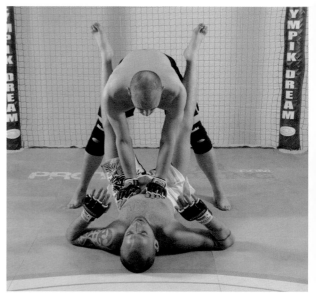

Fig 11.41 The fighter places both hands on to the opponent's stomach and pushes downwards as they straighten their legs.

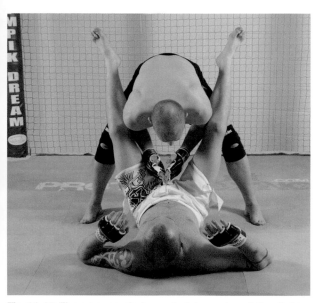

Fig 11.42 The opponent's legs start to part and the fighter tucks their elbows into the inside of their thighs.

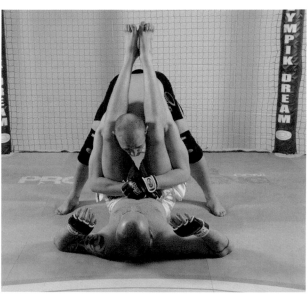

Fig 11.43 The fighter travels around their opponent's legs, capturing and locking the opponent's legs with their arms.

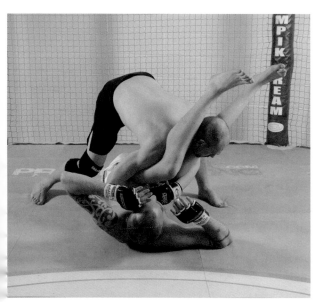

Fig 11.44 The fighter pushes the opponent's legs down to their preferred side.

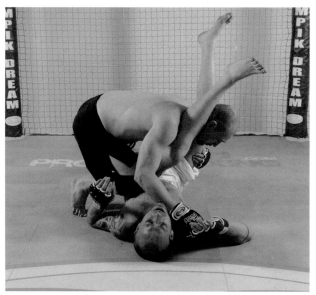

Fig 11.45 The fighter places one hand on their opponent's hip and the other on their shoulder. The knee of the fighter is placed on the opponent's stomach. From this position the fighter has a variety of options, including striking or attempting a submission.

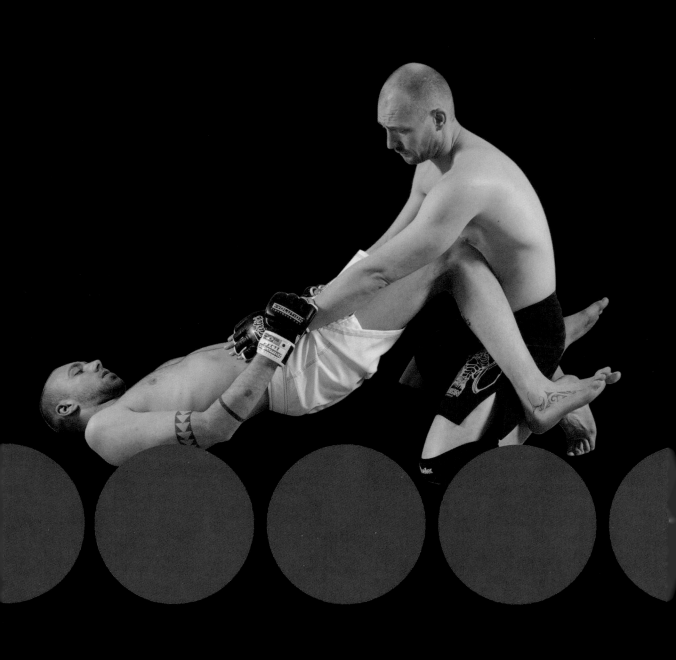

CHAPTER **TWELVE**
Guard bottom

From the guard bottom position a fighter can throw strikes, but as they are unable to put their body weight behind them it's unlikely they will be a threat or generate a knockout. However, this position is advantageous for submissions or sweeps. The opponent should either be held at a distance or very close; anything in between can result in devastating strikes. If the opponent is good on the ground the fighter should also be attempting to return to their feet.

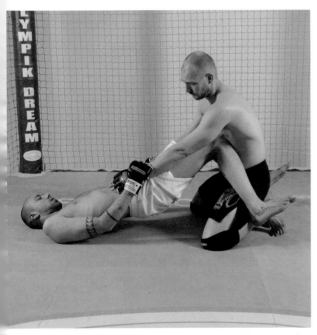

Fig 12.1 The fighter is in the guard bottom position, keeping their opponent out of striking distance.

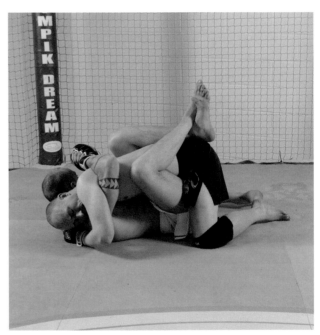

Fig 12.2 The fighter keeps the opponent very close to minimise their striking power.

Sit-up guard to standing

If the opponent's posture is upright, the sit-up guard is an excellent technique for minimising the impact of potentially heavy strikes.

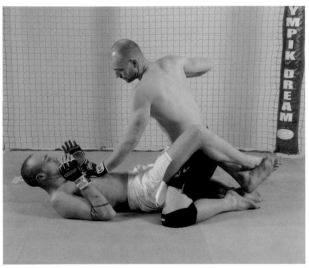

Fig 12.3 The opponent's upright posture places them in a powerful striking position.

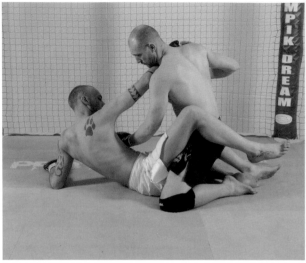

Fig 12.4 To create distance and avoid strikes to the face, the fighter rolls up on to one arm and places the forearm of the other arm on to the opponent's neck.

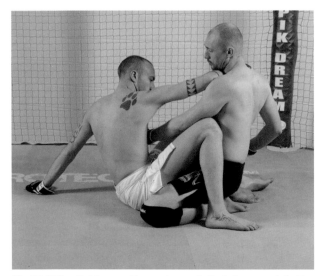

Fig 12.5 The fighter continues to push their forearm into the opponent's neck as they come up on to their hand, locking their elbow, in preparation for pushing up on to their feet.

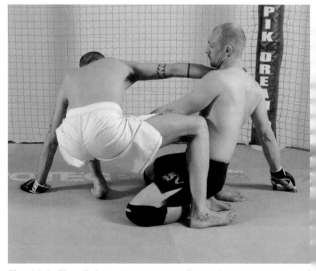

Fig 12.6 The fighter turns away from the opponent and creates space by continuing to push with the hand on their neck.

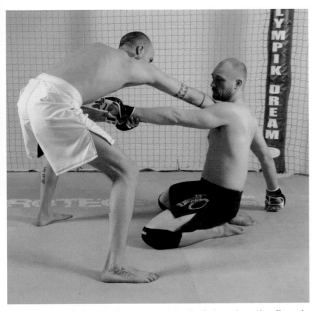

Fig 12.7 The fighter's leg nearest to their hand on the floor is pulled out and placed out of reach of the opponent.

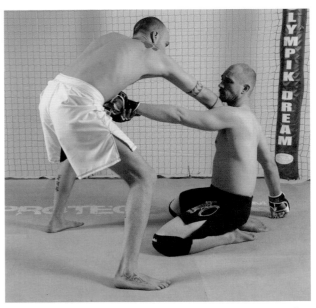

Fig 12.8 The fighter's body is raised while they pull the other leg out of reach. The hand placed on the opponent's neck continues to keep them away.

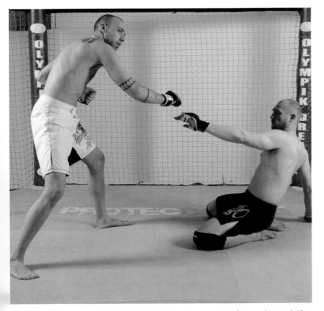

Fig 12.9 Because the fighter's legs are out of reach and the opponent is being pushed away, the opponent is unable to attempt a takedown.

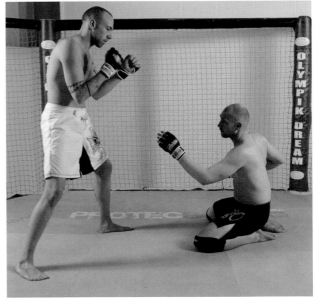

Fig 12.10 The fighter returns to standing.

Hip sweep

The aim of the hip sweep from the guard bottom is to spin the opponent on to their back and secure them in the mount position. The move starts by the fighter moving into the sit-up guard, turning into the opponent and then sweeping them to gain the mount position (the fighter straddling the opponent's abs while the opponent is lying on his back).

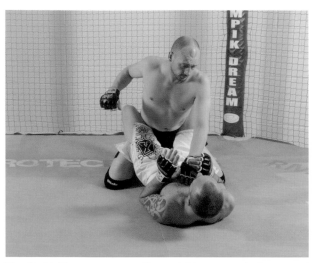

Fig 12.11 The opponent with upright posture is in a good position to land powerful strikes.

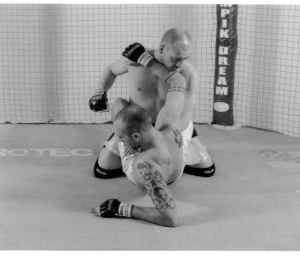

Fig 12.12 To get up, the fighter turns their body to the side and places their non-supporting hand against the opponent's neck.

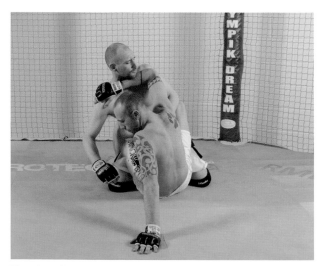

Fig 12.13 The fighter continues to push their forearm into the opponent's neck as they come up from their elbow to their hand.

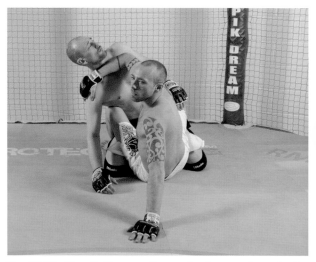

Fig 12.14 The fighter continues to turn and push the opponent's neck to create space.

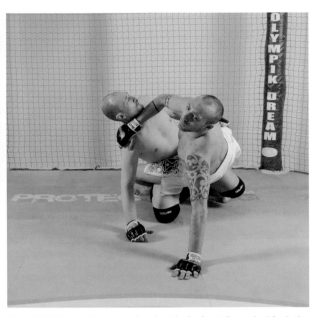

Fig 12.15 The fighter unhooks their feet from behind the opponent's back and continues with their hip now elevated.

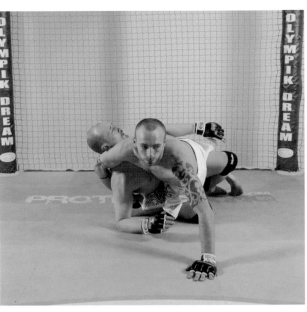

Fig 12.16 The fighter continues to turn their shoulder and hip toward the mat. The arm that was placed on their opponent's neck is now wrapped around their oppenent's arm to prevent a counter sweep.

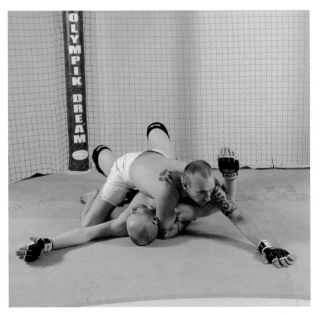

Fig 12.17 With a quick rotation of their hips, the fighter rapidly turns their opponent.

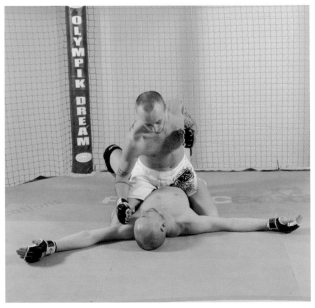

Fig 12.18 The fighter is now in the mount position.

Kimura from guard bottom

This move starts in the same way as the hip sweep, but then differs in response to the opponent placing an arm on the ground and locking their elbow. The fighter then applies the kimura, which involves a lot of pressure on the opponent's shoulder and is therefore likely to create a submission.

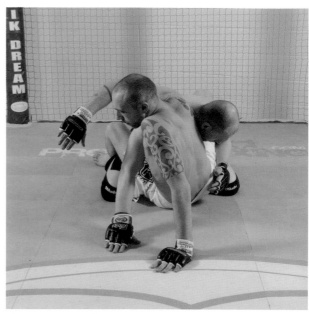

Fig 12.19 The fighter attempts a hip sweep until the opponent counters by placing an arm on the mat.

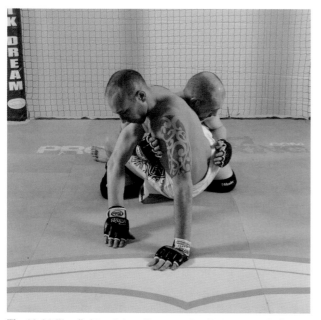

Fig 12.20 The fighter takes the opportunity to wrap their arm around the opponent's arm placed on the mat.

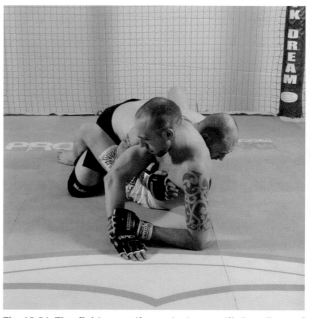

Fig 12.21 The fighter continues to turn until the elbow of their supporting arm is on the mat, at which point the hand of this arm captures the opponent's hand.

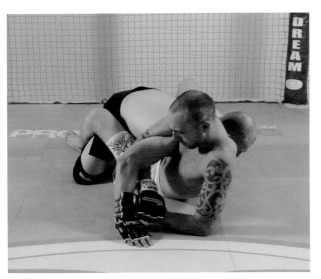

Fig 12.22 The fighter's other hand moves round to join it.

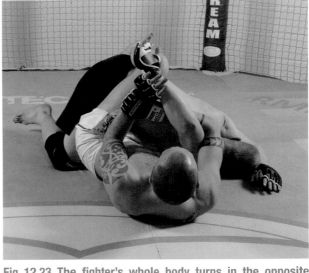

Fig 12.23 The fighter's whole body turns in the opposite direction, this time toward the opponent's head. As the fighter turns on to their back, they place their hip closer to the final position of the kimura to allow for a better angle.

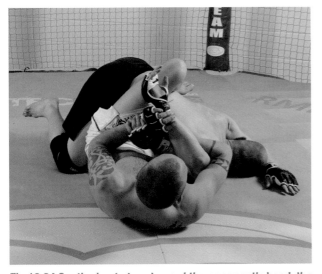

Fig 12.24 Continuing to turn toward the opponent's head, the fighter places their outside leg over the back of the opponent. At the same time, the fighter pulls the arm that is hooked underneath the opponent toward them while pushing the opponent's wrist toward their head. The fighter is now in the kimura position and likely to achieve a submission.

Posture up to a guillotine

The guillotine can be applied when a hip sweep fails due to the opponent countering by lowering their weight into the fighter. The opponent will often lower their head during this move, providing the perfect opportunity to apply the guillotine.

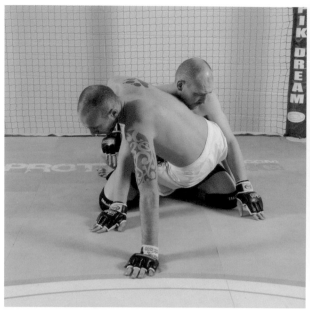

Fig 12.25 The fighter attempts a hip sweep.

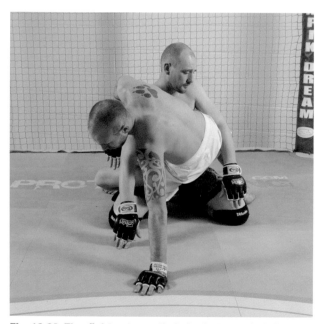

Fig 12.26 The fighter turns their body toward their hand placed on the mat, and at the same time pushes their hips into the opponent.

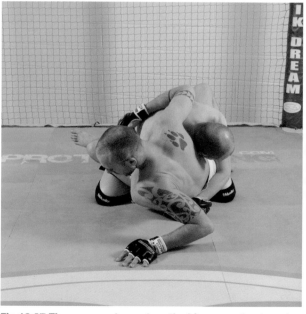

Fig 12.27 The opponent counters the hip sweep by dropping their body down on to the fighter and wrapping their arms around them.

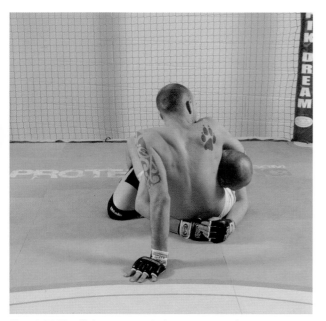

Fig 12.28 The fighter wraps their non-supporting arm around their opponent's head and underneath their chin.

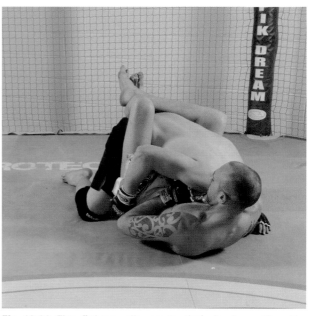

Fig 12.29 The fighter rolls on to their back, pulling the opponent down with them. The fighter's supporting arm is pushed between their bodies to hold the fighter's other wrist.

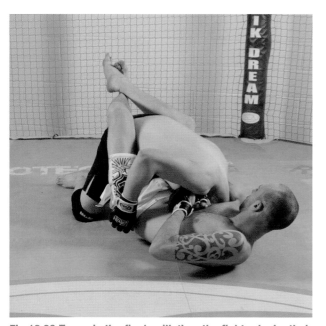

Fig 12.30 To apply the final guillotine, the fighter locks their legs behind the opponent's back and pushes them away, generating even more pressure on their neck.

Arm bar

With the fighter in the sit-up guard, the opponent has reduced options for offensive techniques. One option is to push the fighter back to the ground, however this provides them with the opportunity to apply the arm bar position using the downward force of the opponent.

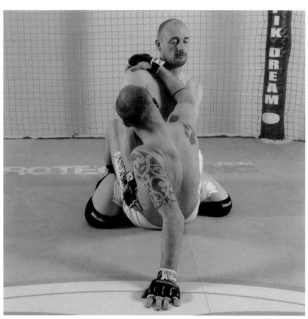 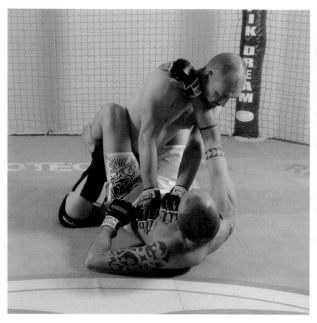

Fig 12.31 The fighter moves into the sit-up guard position by placing their arm on the opponent's neck and pushing up off the elbow of their other arm.

Fig 12.32 The opponent counters by pushing the fighter back to the ground with their hands.

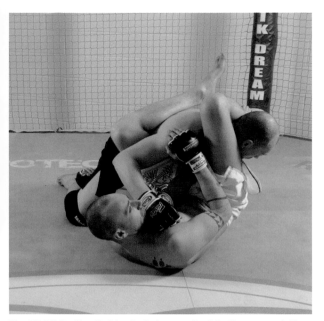

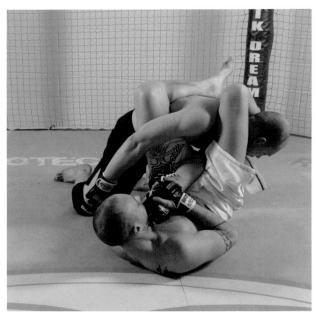

Fig 12.33 As the fighter is being pushed to the ground, they hook their supporting arm around the inside of the opponent's thigh. They then pull their body toward the opponent's thigh and wrap their outside leg over the near side of the opponent's head.

Fig 12.34 The fighter's hand is removed from the opponent's neck as this is now controlled by the fighter's leg. The arm is instead used to pin the opponent's arms to the fighter's chest. For the final part of the move, the fighter raises their hips and applies downward pressure with their legs.

Sit-up guard to back position

When the fighter is in the sit-up guard position they limit their opponent's striking options. The forward momentum of the strikes the opponent makes can be used against them by dodging the blows and capturing the shoulder of the striking arm.

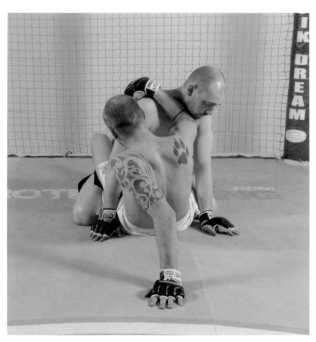

Fig 12.35 The fighter moves into the sit-up guard position by placing their arm on the opponent's neck and supporting themselves with their other hand.

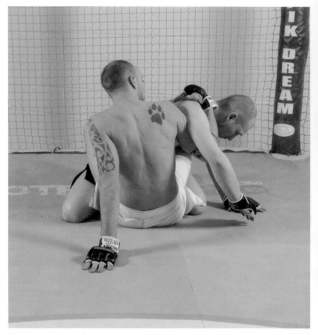

Fig 12.36 The fighter takes the opportunity presented by the opponent attempting to throw an elbow strike to move their head out of the way and capture the opponent's shoulder with the hand that was pushing into their neck.

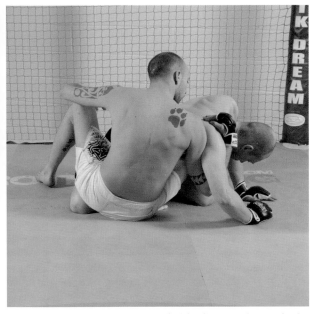

Fig 12.37 The fighter pulls their hip from underneath the opponent by planting their foot and sliding out.

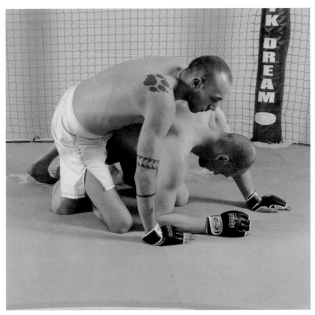

Fig 12.38 The fighter's supporting arm is wrapped around the opponent's back.

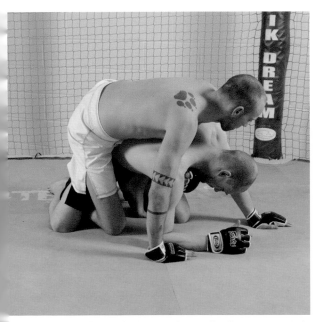

Fig 12.39 The fighter's leg underneath the opponent is placed between their legs.

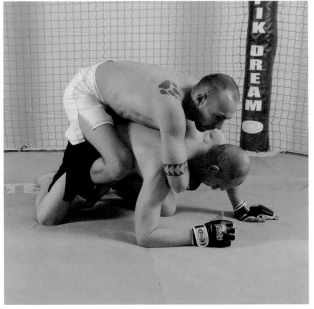

Fig 12.40 The fighter is now in the back mount position with a firm hold.

Getting up from guard bottom

When the fighter is in the guard bottom position with their opponent's head held close, the opponent may attempt to straighten up to create space for them to apply strikes using their body weight. However, the opponent's upward momentum can be used by the fighter to begin to pull themselves back up to standing.

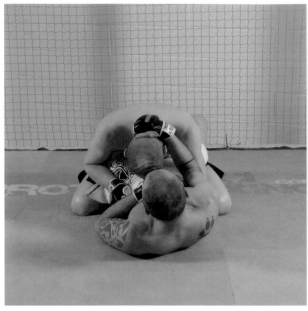

Fig 12.42 The fighter controls the opponent's head from the guard bottom position.

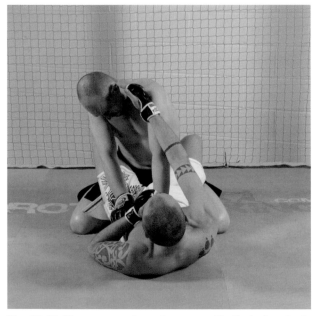

Fig 12.43 The opponent pushes up with their hands to straighten up.

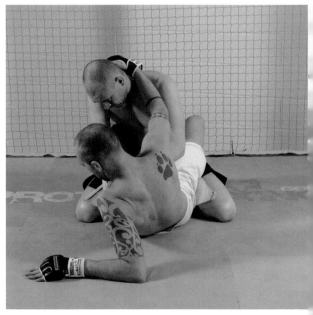

Fig 12.44 The fighter holds on to the opponent's head and uses the upward momentum to roll up on to their other arm.

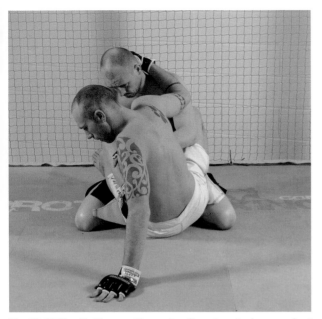

Fig 12.45 The fighter continues to sit up by placing one foot on the mat and moving from the elbow to the hand of the supporting arm.

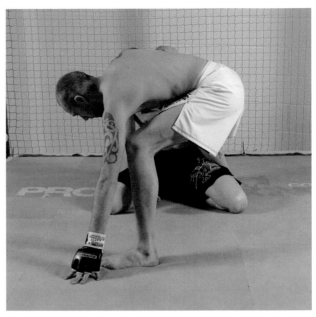

Fig 12.46 The fighter removes their other leg from around the opponent and places it in the back position on the ground. The arm around the opponent's head remains in place to control the distance.

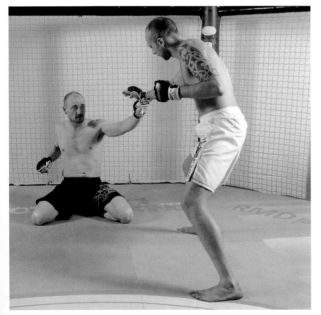

Fig 12.47 The fighter gets up and pushes their opponent away.

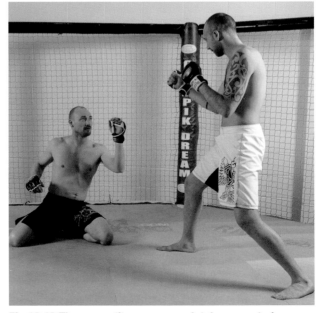

Fig 12.48 The competitors are completely separated.

Elbows from closed guard

Applying strikes while a fighter is on their back is not ideal. However, one of the best strikes from this position is probably the elbow strike. As the opponent's head is close to the fighter's chest in the closed guard position, the fighter has to push their head upward with both hands to create space. The opponent will often try to get their head back to the fighter's body, and when they do the fighter releases their grip and strikes with their elbow.

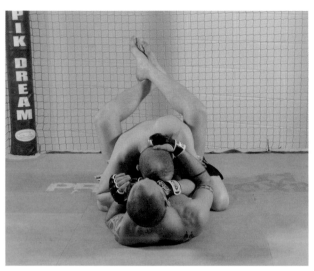

Fig 12.49 The opponent is in the fighter's close guard.

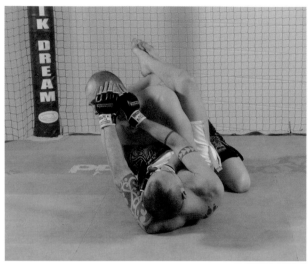

Fig 12.50 The fighter pushes the opponent's head upward to create space.

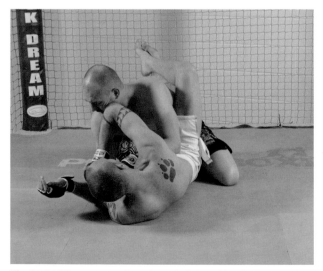

Fig 12.51 The opponent pushes their head back down; when the fighter removes their hands, the opponent's head snaps forwards into the fighter's elbow strike.

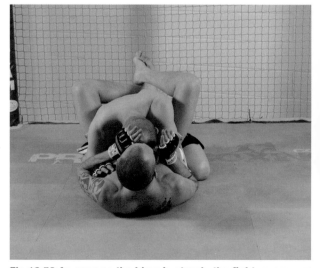

Fig 12.52 As soon as the blow is struck, the fighter removes their arm to prevent it being trapped.

Blocking punches while in guard bottom

The sit-up guard is a good way to hinder an opponent's strikes. However, there are alternatives, including blocking, which work particularly well if the opponent has the fighter pinned to the floor by pushing down on their stomach. At the moment just after the opponent has pulled back their arm to add power to a strike, the fighter combines their forward momentum with a pull forwards of their knees to their chest. The opponent's base is broken, taking power from the punch. Once the opponent's body collapses on to the fighter's body, the fighter has the opportunity to assess their options without being punched.

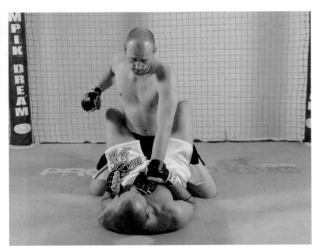

Fig 12.53 The opponent is postured up in the fighter's full guard.

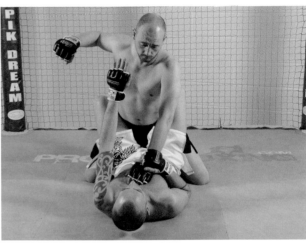

Fig 12.54 The opponent pulls back their striking arm and the fighter protects themselves with their hands.

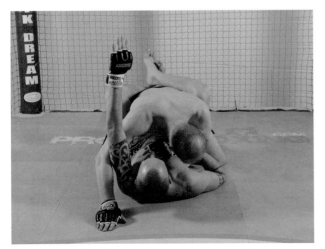

Fig 12.55 The fighter uses the opponent's forward momentum, combined with pulling their knees toward their chest, to intercept the opponent's strike with their arm.

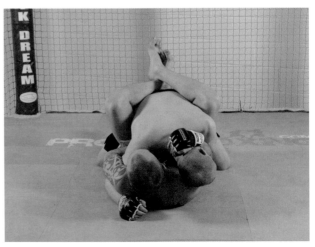

Fig 12.56 The opponent is held down to prevent them from straightening up and delivering another strike.

Another option is to keep one leg behind the opponent's back while the other comes under their shoulder, when they swing back for a strike. During this manoeuvre it is important to maintain the hold on the back of their neck to keep them low.

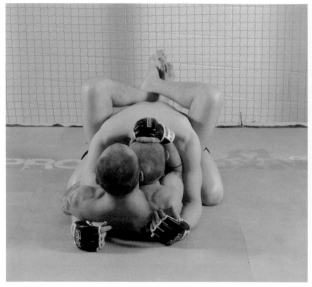

Fig 12.57 The opponent is in the fighter's close guard, with one of the fighter's hands behind their head to prevent them from straightening up and generating additional punch power.

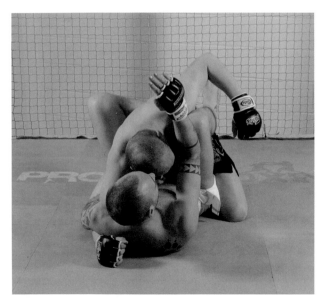

Fig 12.58 The opponent pulls their arm back in preparation for a punch. The fighter places their knee in the shoulder of the opponent's punching arm and lifts their own arm as a block in case their knee doesn't stop the punch.

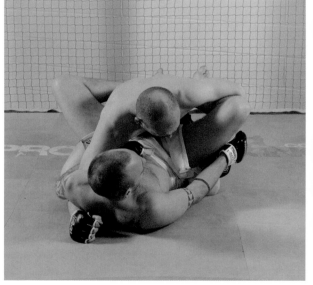

Fig 12.59 The fighter's knee prevents the powerful punch intended for their face. The opponent's head and punching arm are still being controlled by the fighter.

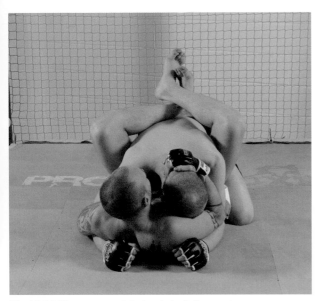

Fig 12.60 The opponent is back in full guard.

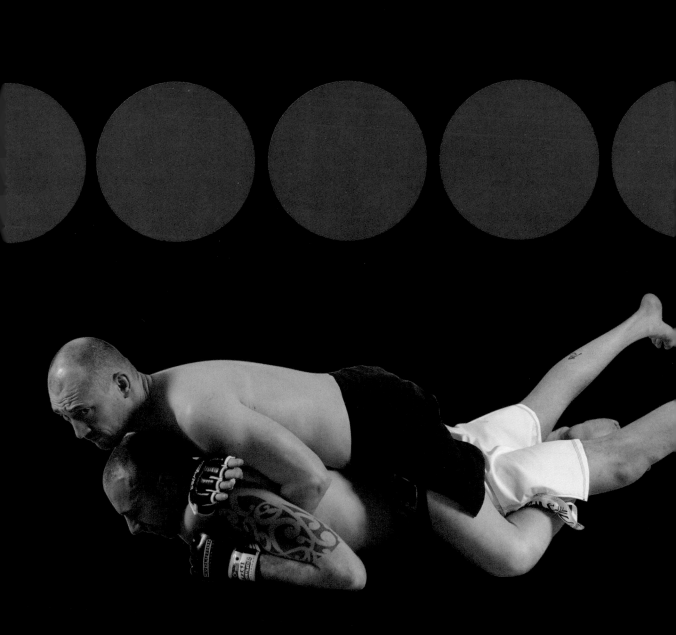

CHAPTER **THIRTEEN**
Half guard top

A *half guard* is when two competitors are on the ground but only one of the fighter's legs is between their opponent's legs. The competitor who is not on their back is described as being in the top position and has many options, although their main objective is to achieve the mount or side control position.

When in the half guard top position it is important to maintain control of the opponent, for example using the under hook around the back of their head. Keeping the opponent pinned flat to the ground is also useful as it prevents them from executing a sweep.

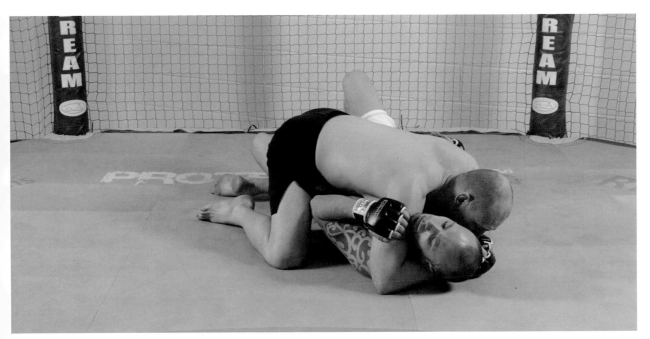

Fig 13.1 Half guard top.

Half guard top to pass to mount

By passing from the half guard into the mount, the fighter places themselves in a more advantageous position for strikes. During the transition the fighter controls their opponent's head and one of their arms as this minimises their ability to punch. The fighter also has to keep their head low and their hips high to escape their opponent's leg hold. Once their foot is free, they can go for the mount position.

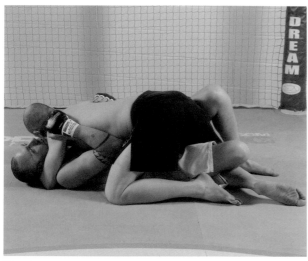

Fig 13.2 The fighter in the opponent's half guard is controlling the opponent's head and one of their arms.

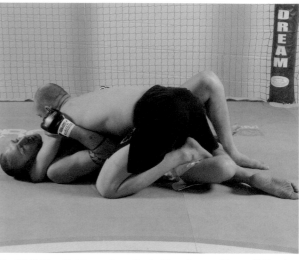

Fig 13.3 The fighter raises their hips by pushing off the leg that is between the opponent's. Their other foot is placed on their opponent's knee.

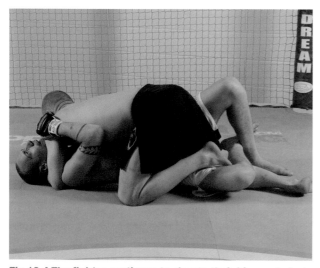

Fig 13.4 The fighter continues to elevate their hips and starts pushing their shoulder into their opponent's face.

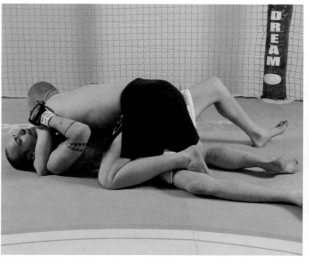

Fig 13.5 The fighter forces their opponent's knee to the ground with their foot.

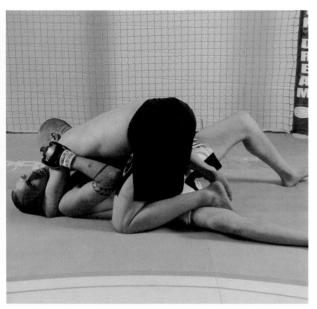

Fig 13.6 The fighter's legs pin one of the opponent's legs to the ground and start to wedge the other leg by placing one knee over the opponent's thigh.

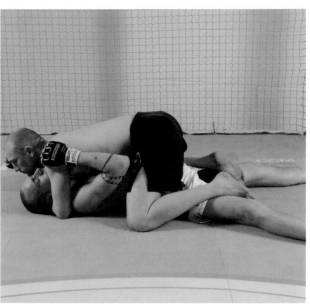

Fig 13.7 The fighter straddles the opponent's hips and flattens their whole body on to their opponent's.

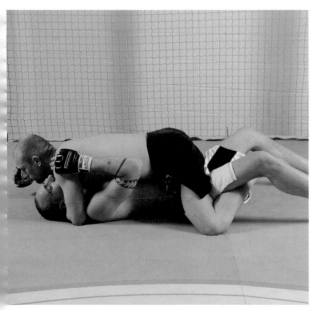

Fig 13.8 The fighter secures the mount by wrapping their legs underneath their opponent's and placing their heels together.

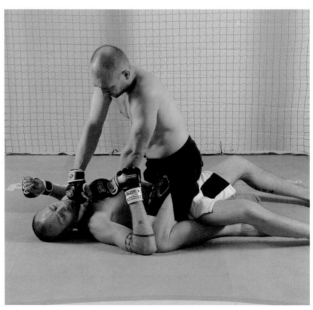

Fig 13.9 The fighter throws a punch from the mount position.

Half guard bottom

It is important for the fighter to quickly get out of this position as they are more likely to be struck by their opponent and they themselves have limited strike options. The fighter needs to move about as much as possible to put their opponent off balance and to create opportunities to adopt new positions.

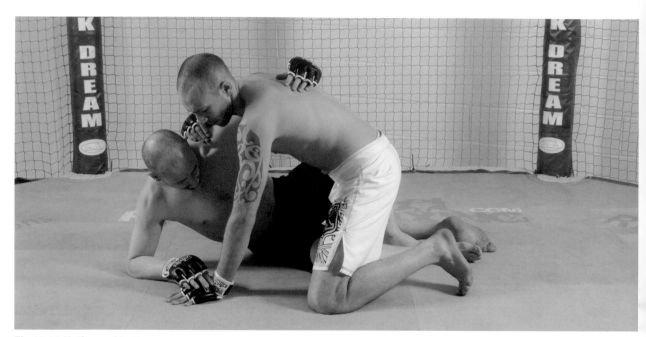

Fig 13.10 Half guard bottom.

Half guard bottom to back

The fighter on the bottom aims to get out of this position by hooking their opponent's legs and, if the opponent doesn't try to counter with an over hook, twisting their body into their opponent's, forcing them to put a hand to the ground for balance. The fighter then quickly twists his body and works around the opponent's back.

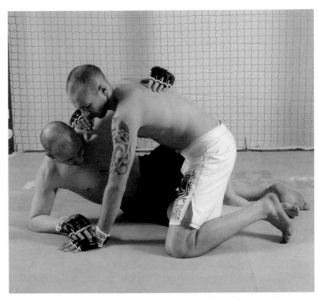

Fig 13.11 The opponent is in the fighter's half guard.

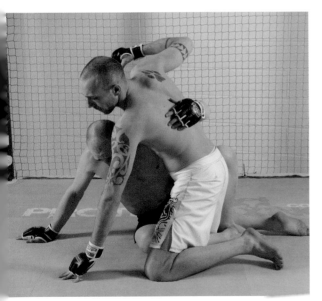

Fig 13.12 The opponent straightens up to strike and the fighter takes the opportunity to turn into the opponent.

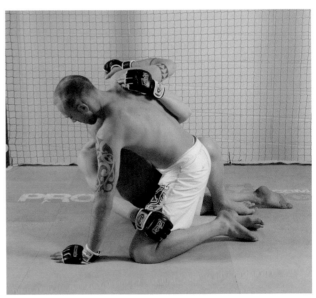

Fig 13.13 The fighter separates their legs and places one foot on the mat. The arm on the fighter's free side is wrapped around the opponent's leg, which is between theirs. The fighter's other arm hooks underneath the opponent's other leg. The opponent is forced off balance and therefore places a hand on the ground for support.

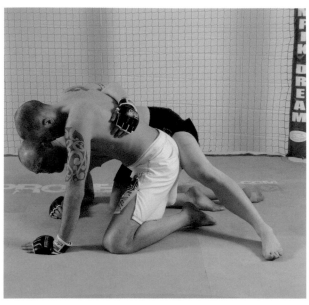

Fig 13.14 The fighter turns both their body and that of their opponent, and places their leg over their opponent's leg, which is between theirs.

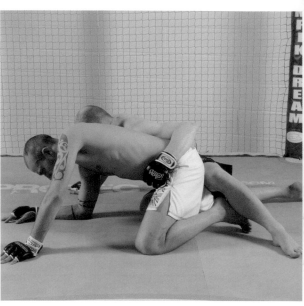

Fig 13.15 The fighter hooks the opponent's leg and pulls back while maintaining a firm hold of the opponent's hips.

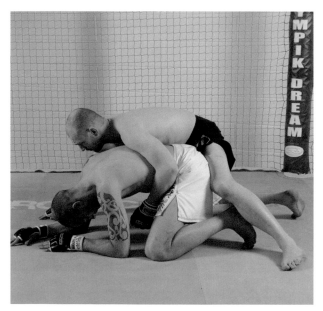

Fig 13.16 The fighter releases their hold on their opponent's inside leg, pushing the opponent off base, turning and coming up on to their elbow.

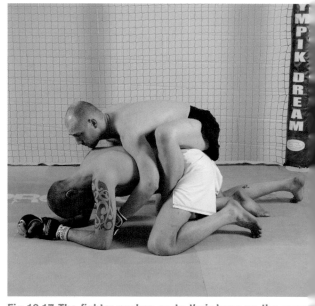

Fig 13.17 The fighter pushes on to their knee on the same side while continuing to rotate on to their opponent's back. The supporting leg is wrapped around the front of the opponent's thigh as the other is launched over their back.

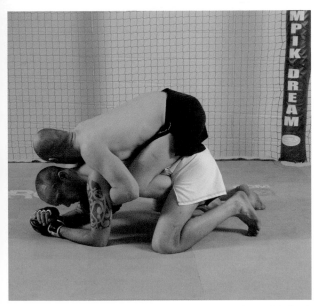

Fig 13.18 The fighter secures the back position with both legs wrapped around the inside of their opponent's legs. The fighter is in a very strong position with several options open.

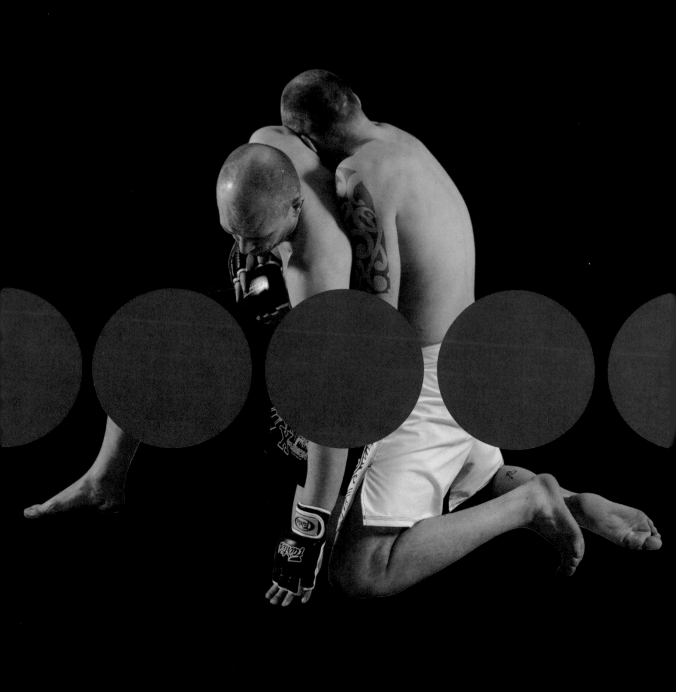

CHAPTER **FOURTEEN**
Side control

In the side control position the fighter lays their torso on top of their opponent's while locking their arms around their neck. To be effective, the fighter must push their body weight down on to their opponent while lowering their hips to the ground.

This is a transition position because to apply powerful punches the fighter has to free their hands and gain height.

Punching and elbowing from standard side control

To execute an effective strike, the fighter has to gain height by escaping the opponent's arm lock, while also controlling their arms. In this example, the fighter uses their knee on the opponent's bicep, which also leaves their opponent's head unprotected.

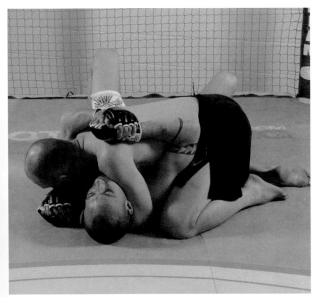

Fig 14.1 The fighter is in the standard side control position, with one arm around the opponent's neck and the other hooked underneath their arm. To protect themselves, the opponent closes the space between by locking their arms around the fighter's back.

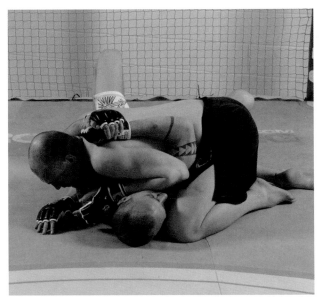

Fig 14.2 The fighter releases their arm from the opponent's neck and places their forearm on their face.

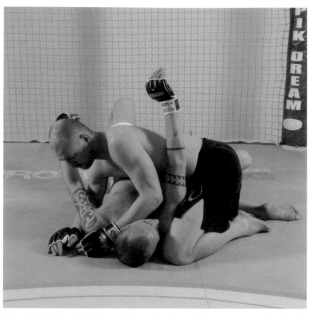

Fig 14.3 The fighter drives their wrist down on to their opponent's jaw, forcing their head to the side and their hands apart.

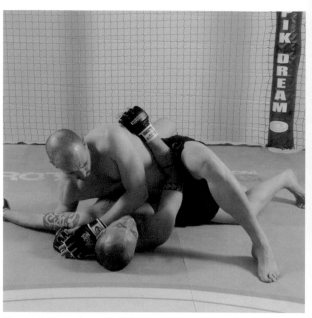

Fig 14.4 The released fighter turns their torso toward their opponent's head and comes up on to their front foot.

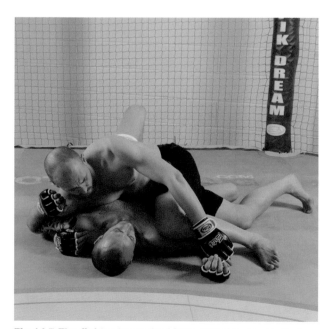

Fig 14.5 The fighter traps the bicep of their opponent's free arm with their hand, and brings their front knee forwards.

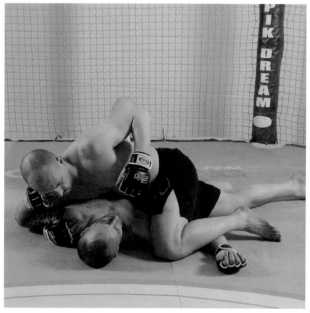

Fig 14.6 The fighter's knee is placed over the opponent's bicep, which is pinned to the mat with the fighter's shin.

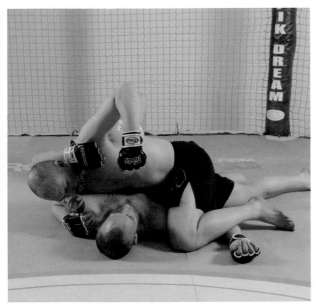

Fig 14.7 Both of the opponent's arms are controlled, one behind the fighter's neck and the other pinned to the floor by the fighter's shin. The fighter now has a choice of strikes.

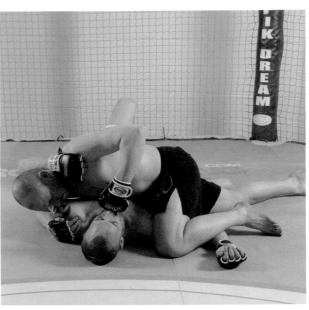

Fig 14.8 The fighter punches the opponent's face with their free arm.

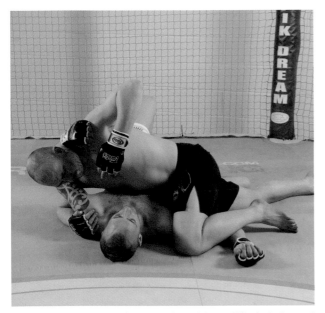

Fig 14.9 The opponent is very vulnerable and likely to tap out or be knocked out. The fighter prepares for a second blow to their face.

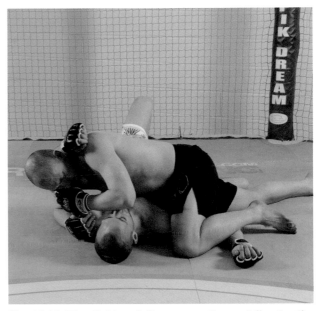

Fig 14.10 The fighter delivers an elbow strike to the opponent's unprotected face.

Americana from side control

To increase the effectiveness of submission techniques, it is important to include distracting strikes in the set-up. In the Americana the fighter traps one arm so the opponent is forced to defend their face with the other. However, the vulnerability created by the movement to defend is used by the fighter as they capture the defending arm and apply the submission.

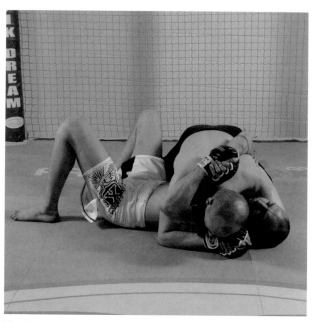

Fig 14.17 The fighter is in the side control position.

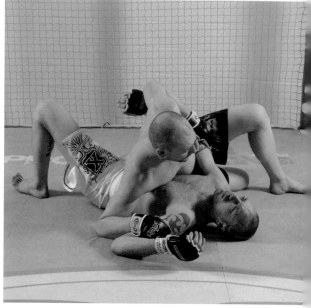

Fig 14.18 The fighter moves to face their opponent by turning their torso toward them. The fighter's arm on the mat is firmly placed next to their opponent's hip while also securing their elbow. The other hand is placed on the inside of their opponent's other arm, which they begin to push between their legs.

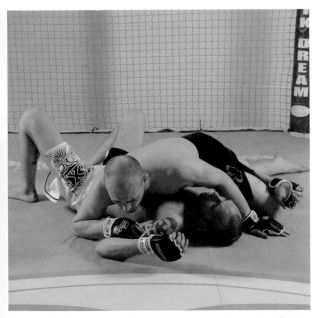

Fig 14.19 The opponent's arm is trapped by the fighter squeezing their knees together.

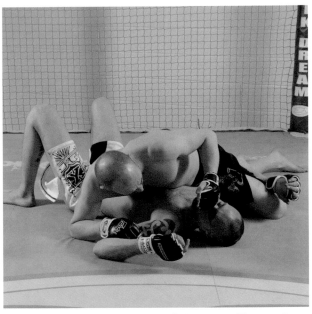

Fig 14.20 From this position, the fighter can either apply an elbow or hammer fist to their opponent's face. In this example a hammer fist is shown.

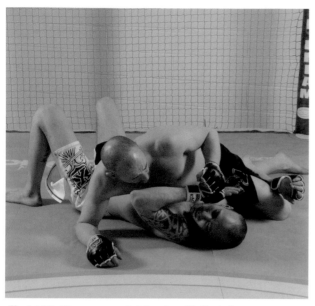

Fig 14.21 The opponent defends with their free arm.

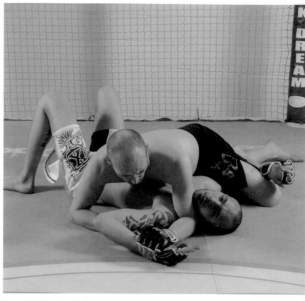

Fig 14.22 The fighter captures the wrist of the defending arm with their striking hand. The fighter's other hand is placed near the opponent's shoulder.

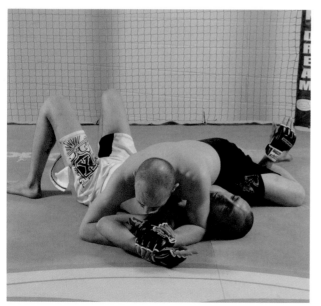

Fig 14.23 The fighter puts all their body weight on to the opponent by turning and lowering their hips. The opponent's arm is held and pushed toward the floor between the fighter's arms.

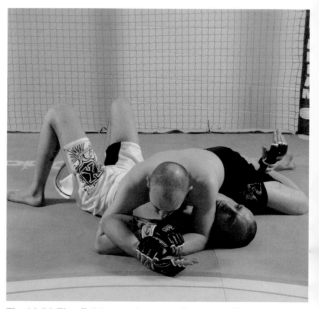

Fig 14.24 The fighter captures and secures the opponent's wrist closest to the ground.

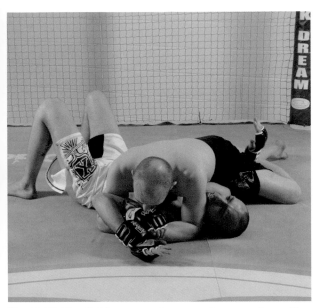

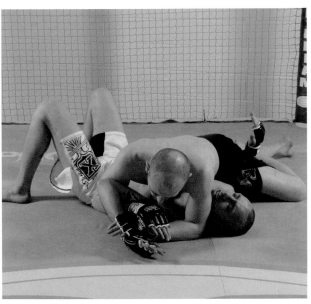

Fig 14.25 The fighter generates more leverage by pulling both their elbows toward the opponent's body.

Fig 14.26 The opponent's arm is twisted by pulling their elbow up and pushing their wrist down. The twist is applied until they submit.

Side control to mount

Because the mount position provides good opportunities for striking, the opponent tries to prevent the fighter from achieving it by crossing their legs. The fighter deals with this by pushing their opponent's top knee toward the ground with their hand to create space for their leg to move over.

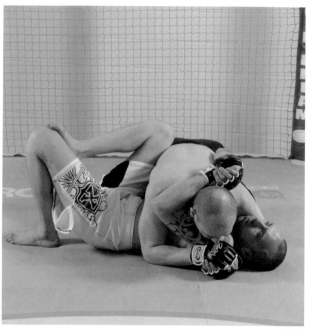

Fig 14.27 The fighter is in the side control position.

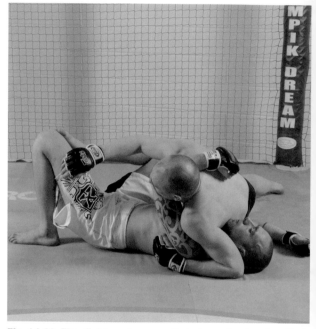

Fig 14.28 The fighter changes their base by turning their torso toward their opponent's legs.

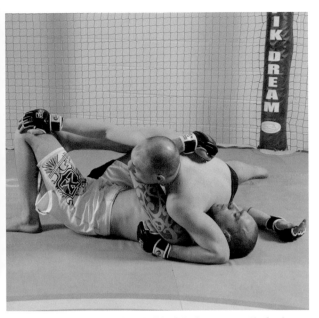

Fig 14.29 The fighter takes hold of their opponent's far knee.

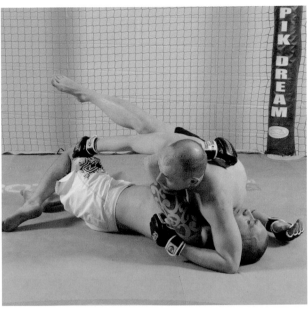

Fig 14.30 The opponent's knee is pushed toward the ground to create space for the fighter's leg to go over the opponent's body.

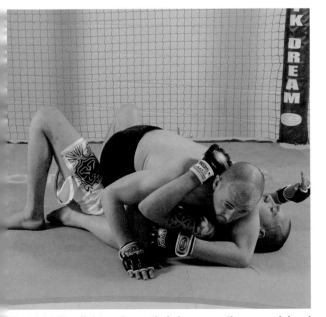

Fig 14.31 The fighter places their knees on the ground, level with the opponent's hips. To secure the position, the fighter brings their heels together underneath the opponent's legs.

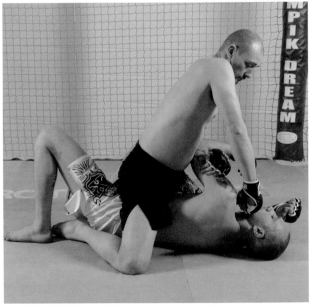

Fig 14.32 The fighter straightens up and prepares to punch.

161

Side control to knee on stomach

If it has not been possible to achieve the mount position, the fighter has the option of placing their knee on the opponent's stomach to gain height and therefore more striking options.

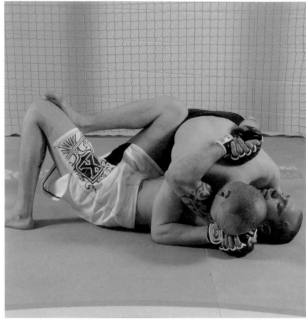

Fig 14.33 The fighter is in the side control position.

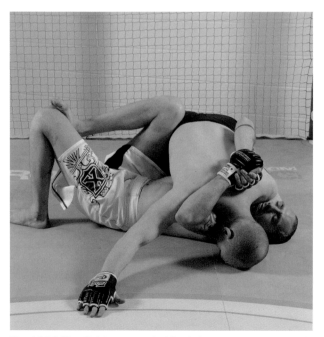

Fig 14.34 The fighter extends his right arm and places his forehead on the ground.

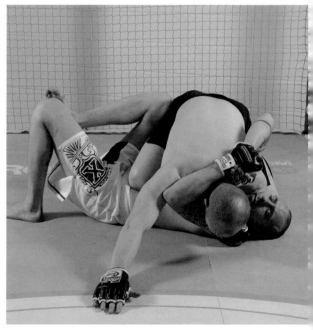

Fig 14.35 The fighter uses the head and the extended arm for leverage in order to place the knee on the stomach.

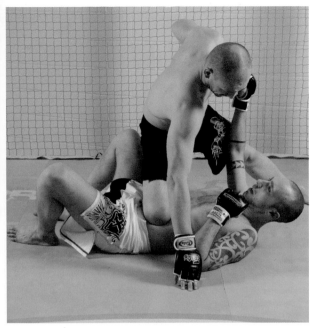

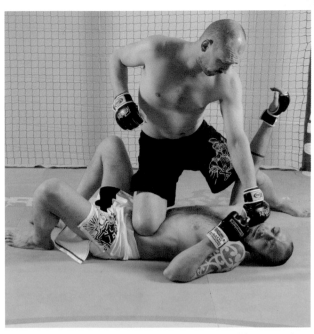

Fig 14.36 The fighter comes up on his knee to pull back his striking arm.

Fig 14.37 The fighter strikes their opponent with a punch.

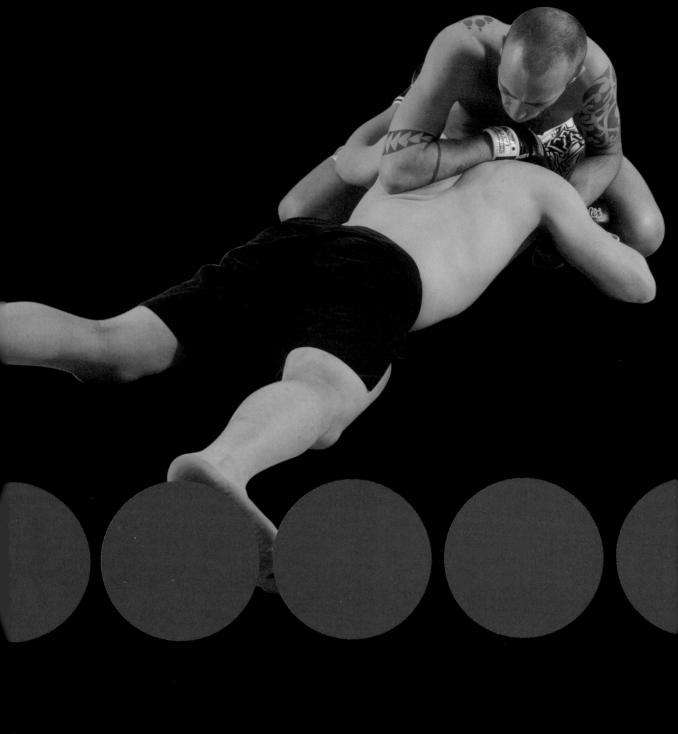

CHAPTER FIFTEEN
Defence against side control

It is essential for the fighter to learn how to escape from an opponent's side control as it places them in a very vulnerable position.

Side control to full guard

The fighter turns into their opponent and pushes on their outside leg to move their hips away from the opponent. The gap created is maintained by pushing their hands against their opponent's hips. The fighter's non-supporting leg passes between their bodies, again to maintain the gap created. The supporting leg is wrapped around the opponent's back and the full guard is applied by the fighter placing one hand around their opponent's neck.

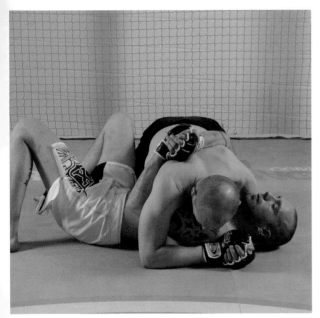

Fig 15.1 The fighter is held in the side control position.

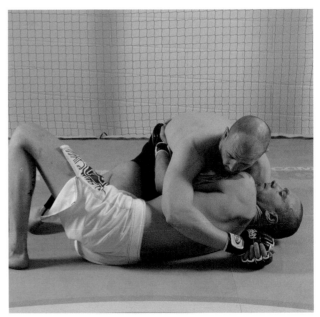

Fig 15.2 The fighter turns their torso toward their opponent, placing their foot on the ground to push their hips away and maintaining the gap by placing both their hands on their opponent's hips.

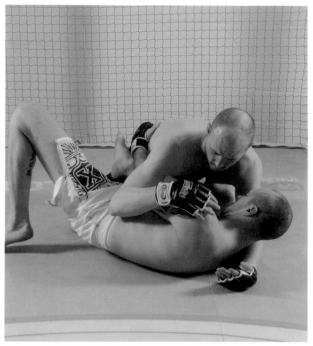

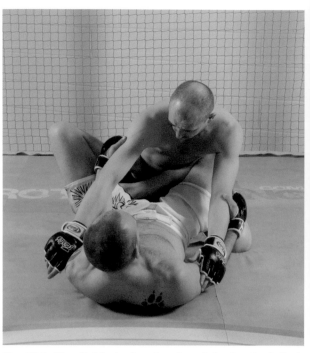

Fig 15.3 The fighter's leg nearest to their opponent travels between their bodies to help maintain the gap.

Fig 15.4 The fighter's leg is placed in front of their opponent's hips.

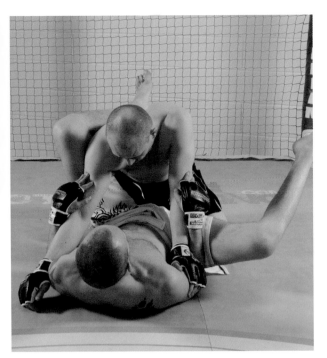

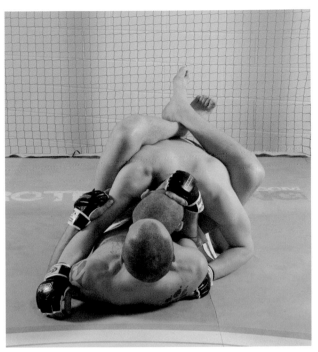

Fig 15.5 The fighter's supporting leg is wrapped around their opponent's back, while the other is pulled clear.

Fig 15.6 Once clear, this leg is also wrapped around the opponent's back. The opponent's posture is controlled by placing an arm around their neck.

Side control to standing

The fighter slides away from their opponent on to their stomach, knees and finally their feet.

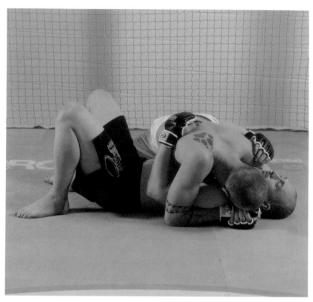

Fig 15.7 The fighter is held in the side control position.

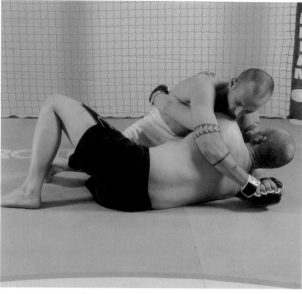

Fig 15.8 The fighter turns into their opponent and pushes their hips with their hands to move themselves away.

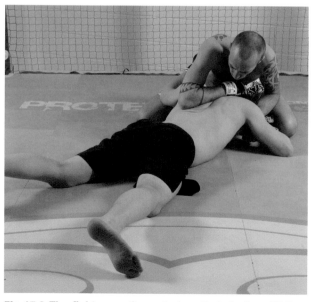

Fig 15.9 The fighter continues to turn their body until they are facing down on the mat.

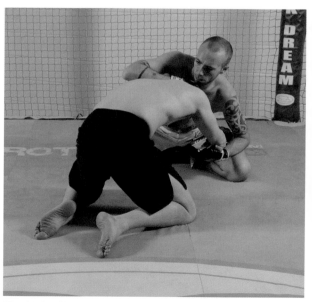

Fig 15.10 The fighter quickly moves onto their knees to prevent the opponent taking their back.

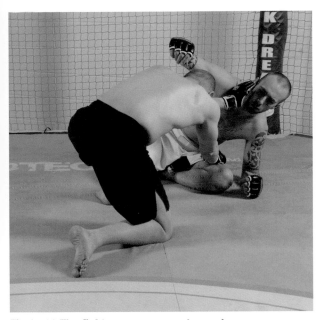

Fig 15.11 The fighter comes up on to one leg.

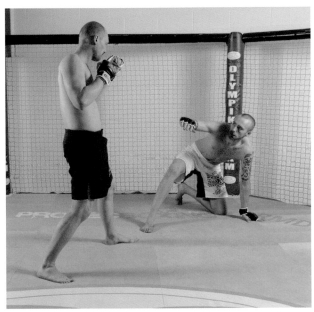

Fig 15.12 The fighter is now back on his feet.

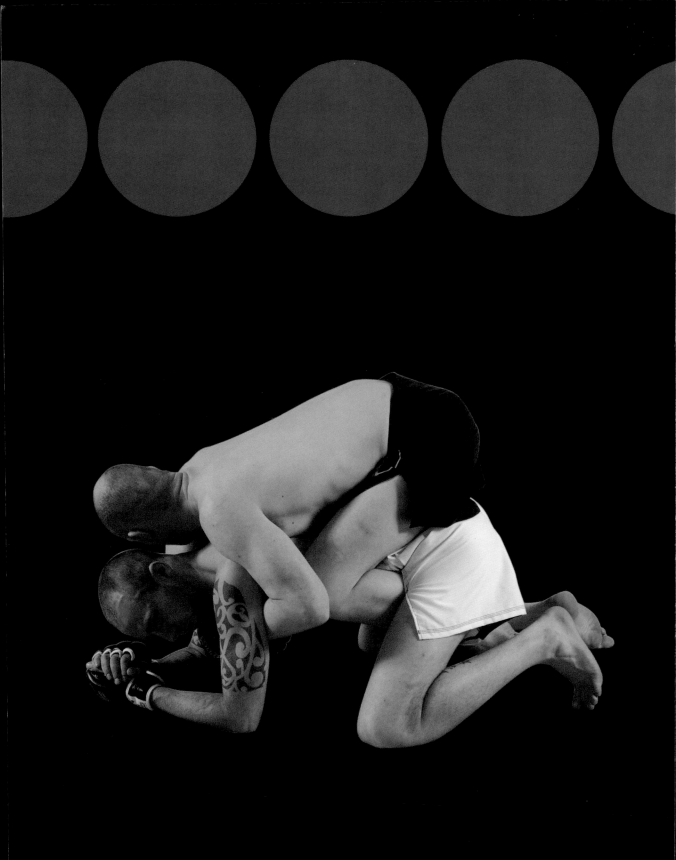

CHAPTER **SIXTEEN**
Attacking techniques when taking an opponent's back

Correctly applying the back position creates one of the most dominant positions in MMA as there is little the opponent can do in defence. The opponent will therefore try everything to not be caught in this way.

Turtle to back position

The fighter initially secures the turtle position by lowering their weight on to their opponent's back and hooking one arm around their body. The fighter's inside knee is placed very close and parallel to the opponent's body while standing on their other leg to provide extra stability.

The opponent has their elbows close to their knees in a defensive position to prevent the fighter from achieving a leg hook. To move the opponent's elbows, the fighter strikes their head with a punch. As the opponent protects themselves with their arm, the fighter applies their first leg hook, turns the opponent on to their back and then applies a choke.

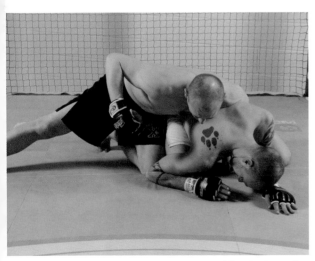

Fig 16.1 The fighter secures the turtle position by lowering their weight on to their opponent's lower back and hooking their arm around them. The fighter's inside knee is placed parallel to the opponent's body and extra stability is gained by having the outside foot on the ground. The fighter's free arm is pulled back in preparation to apply a punch.

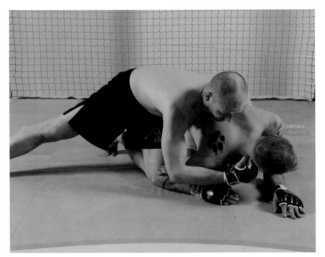

Fig 16.2 The fighter applies a strike to the opponent's face while keeping their elbows in a leg hook defence position close to their knees.

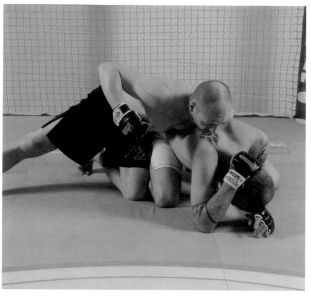

Fig 16.3 The opponent brings their arm toward their head to protect against another strike to the face.

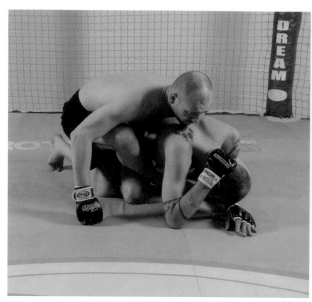

Fig 16.4 The fighter takes the opportunity created to slide their outside foot inside and around the opponent's hip to secure the first hook.

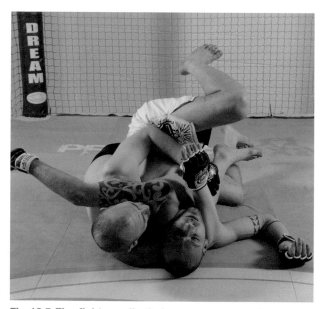

Fig 16.5 The fighter pulls their opponent toward them and wraps their free arm around their neck.

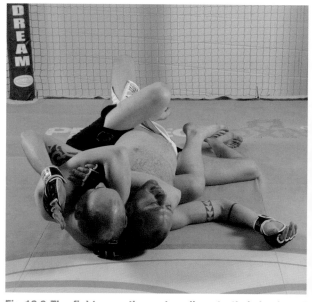

Fig 16.6 The fighter continues to roll on to their back and secures their second leg hook. The fighter applies a choke hold by placing one arm around their opponent's neck, the other on their head, and squeezing their arms together.

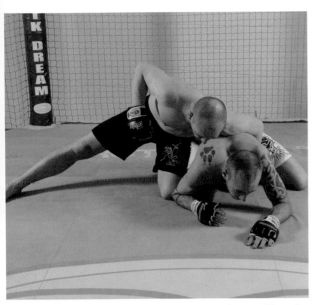

Fig 16.7 The fighter secures the turtle position by distributing their weight over the opponent's lower back and wrapping one arm around their body.

Preventing an opponent from countering the back position

With the opponent in the turtle position, and the fighter in the secured back position with their legs hooked around the inside of their opponent's legs, the opponent has to stand up and shake them off before they can apply any other techniques. To prevent this, the fighter wraps their arm around the leg the opponent is trying to stand on.

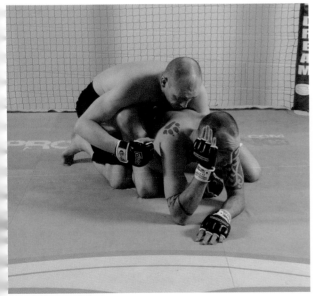

Fig 16.8 The fighter strikes their opponent's head, forcing them to defend. By bringing their elbow forward, the opponent creates a space that the fighter uses to apply their first leg hook.

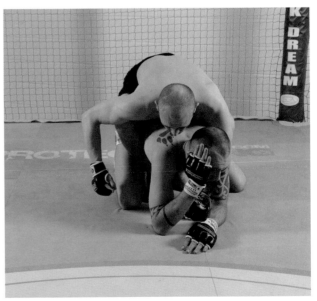

Fig 16.9 The second hook is applied by the fighter bringing their other leg over their opponent's body.

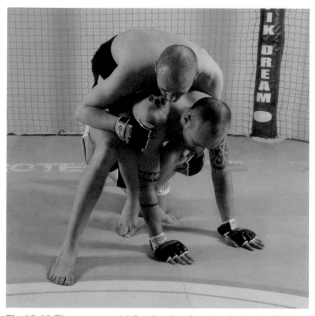

Fig 16.10 The opponent tries to stand up to shake the fighter off their back by pushing up on to their hands and one leg.

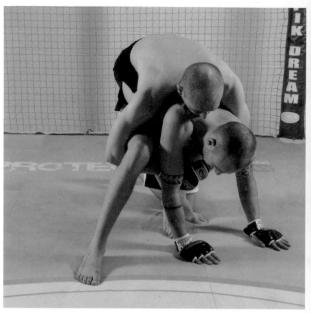

Fig 16.11 The moment the opponent comes up on to one foot, the fighter catches their leg by wrapping their arm around it, effectively preventing them from standing up any further.

Flattening the opponent in the turtle position

With the opponent in the turtle position and the fighter in the back control position, the fighter pushes their opponent's body flat to the ground. This is achieved by the fighter wrapping their legs around their opponent's hips, pushing back with their legs and toward the ground with their hips. Once the opponent is flat, the fighter can either apply punches or a choke hold.

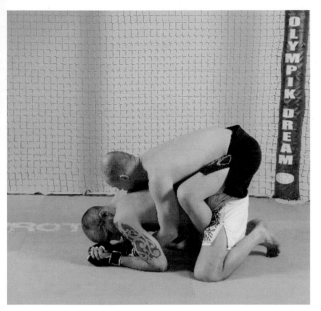

Fig 16.12 The fighter secures the back control position by wrapping both their legs around their opponent's hips and their arms around the opponent's chest.

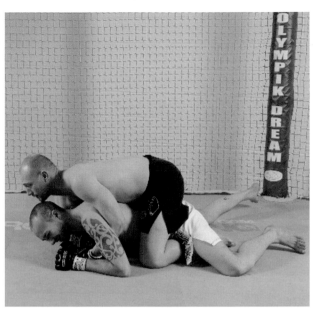

fig 16.13 The fighter pushes their legs back and their hips toward the ground.

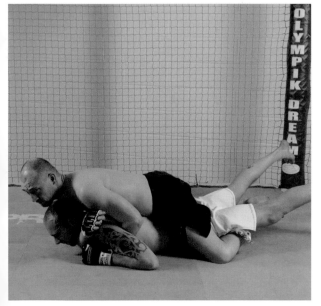

Fig 16.14 While the opponent is flat on the mat, the fighter straightens as they continue to push their hips toward the ground.

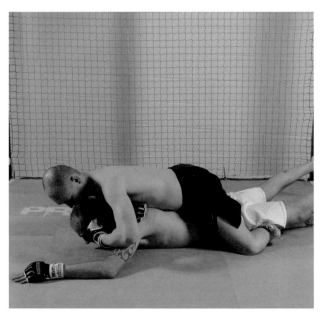

Fig 16.15 The fighter applies punches to the side of their opponent's head.

Arm bar from back control position

When seated, the fighter has their opponent in the back position with both feet placed on their inner thigh. By turning their body toward where the arm bar will be applied, the fighter places their leg from the same side on their opponent's hip. The other leg is placed over the opponent's head and the arm bar applied with the opponent's thumb pointing to the ceiling.

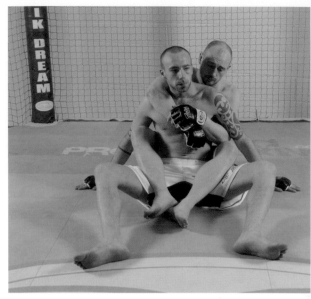

Fig 16.16 The fighter sits behind their opponent with their feet on their opponent's inner thigh.

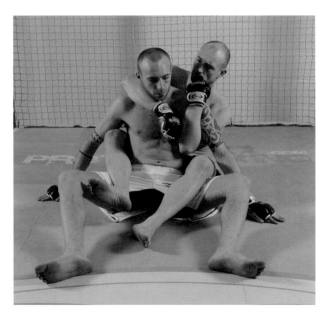

Fig 16.17 The fighter pivots toward the side where the arm bar will be applied and also places their foot on their opponent's outer hip to assist with the movement. The fighter holds the arm to which the arm bar will be applied.

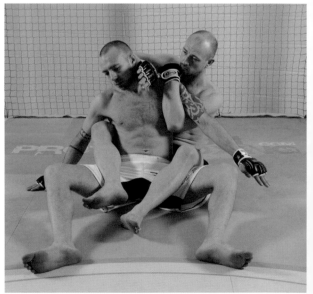

Fig 16.18 While continuing to rotate, the fighter slips their other arm over the opponent's head.

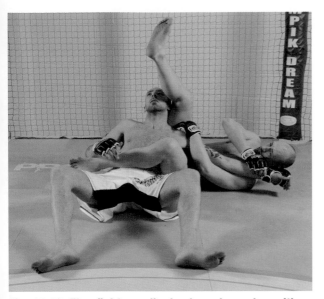

Fig 16.19 The fighter rolls backwards and positions themselves at a 90-degree angle to their opponent's body. A leg is also placed over the opponent's lower body to prevent them from straightening up.

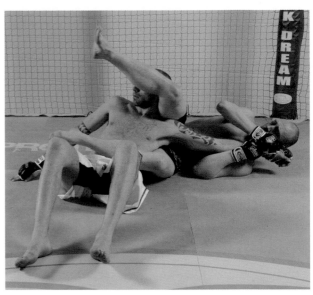

Fig 16.20 The fighter pulls their other leg from underneath their opponent's body and places it over the opponent's head.

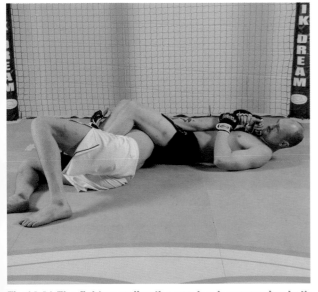

Fig 16.21 The fighter applies the arm bar by squeezing both their knees together, elevating their hips and pulling the opponent's arm toward their chest with their thumb pointing upwards.

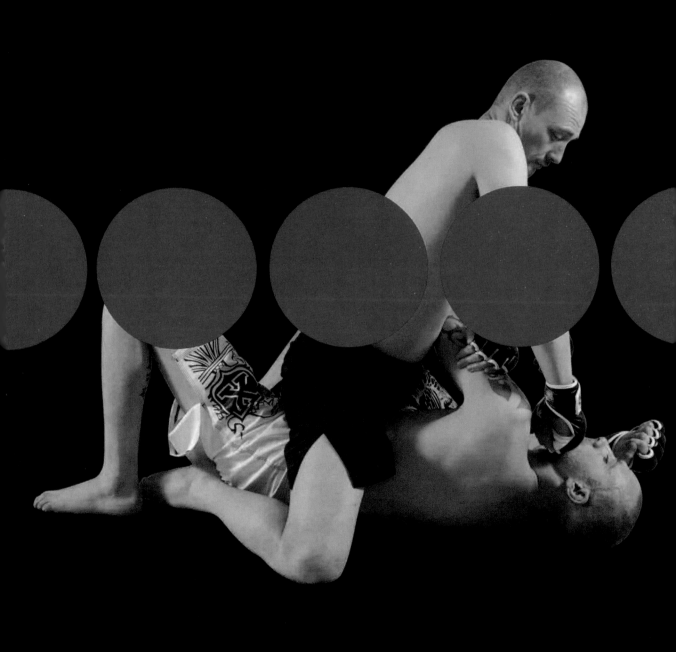

CHAPTER **SEVENTEEN**
Defence against back control

When the fighter's back is being attacked they are at a disadvantage and therefore should escape as quickly as possible.

Escaping the turtle position by standing up

A fighter in the turtle position with their opponent applying an under hook body lock counters the move by coming up on to one and then both feet. Once standing, they wedge their thumbs into the top of their opponent's hands and push the hands toward the ground. At the same time, the fighter leans into their opponent, but pushes their hips forward and steps away. The fighter then turns toward their opponent and assumes the fighting stance.

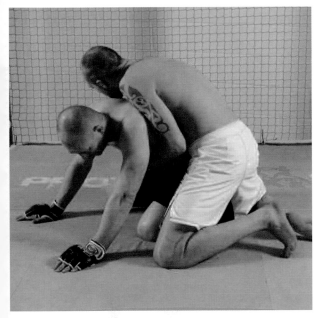

Fig 17.1 The opponent holds the fighter in a double under hook body lock in the turtle position.

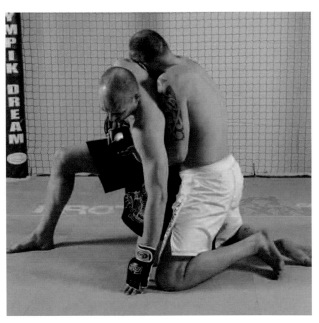

Fig 17.2 The fighter quickly gets up on to one foot.

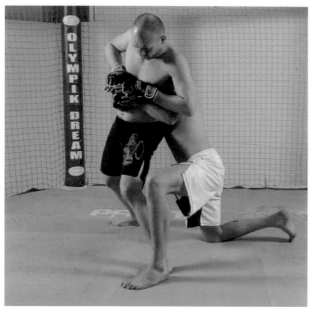

Fig 17.3 The fighter is back on both feet and starts to wedge their thumbs into the top of their opponent's hands.

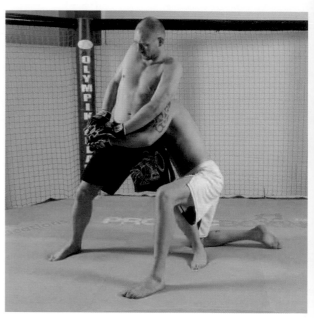

Fig 17.4 The fighter steps forward with their front leg, leaning their upper body back and pushing their hips forward while also pushing their opponent's hands down.

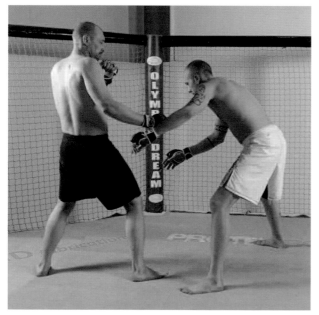

Fig 17.5 The fighter breaks their opponent's grip and continues to turn away from them.

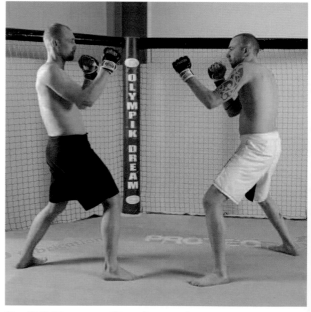

Fig 17.6 The competitors face each other in the fighting stance.

Choke defence from back control

When the fighter is being held in the back control position their opponent is likely to apply a choke hold. To protect against this, the fighter should prevent access to their neck by using, for example, the figure four defence position.

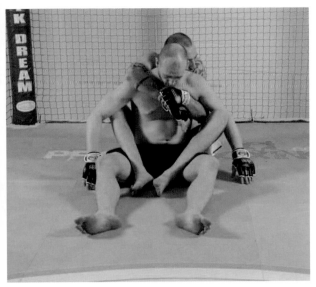

Fig 17.7 The fighter is being held in the back control position with their opponent's feet around their hips.

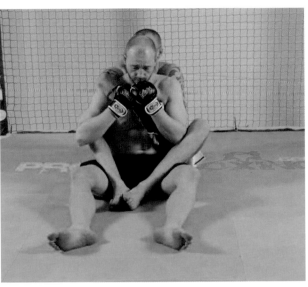

Fig 17.8 The fighter brings up their hands to protect their neck.

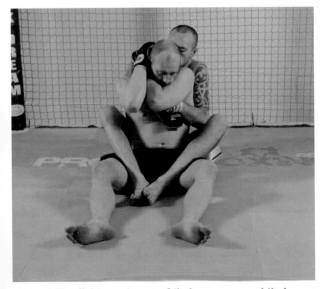

Fig 17.9 The fighter puts one of their arms around their own neck and coils the other arm around it.

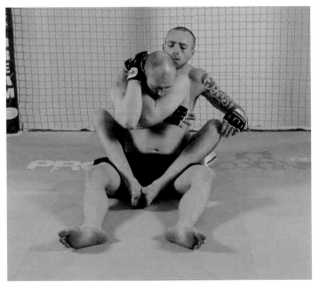

Fig 17.10 The opponent tries unsuccessfully to find a gap.

181

Bottom turtle into guard

The fighter uses a forward roll toward their opponent to remove them from their back and to obtain the more advantageous guard position. The technique is most effective when the opponent hasn't established hooks and therefore doesn't have total control of the fighter's back.

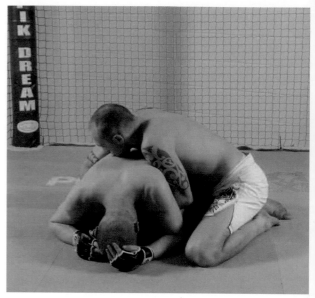

Fig 17.11 The opponent has their arms wrapped around the fighter's lower back while they are in the turtle position.

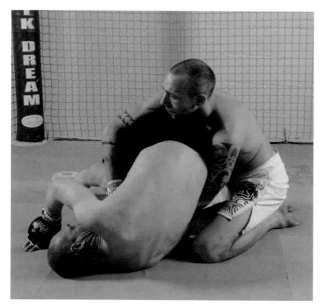

Fig 17.12 Before the opponent secures leg hooks, the fighter reacts by rolling forward on to their shoulder closest to their opponent. This also has the effect of moving their hips away from their opponent's body.

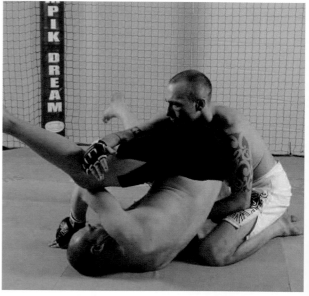

Fig 17.13 The fighter continues to roll forward, making it difficult for their opponent to maintain their hold.

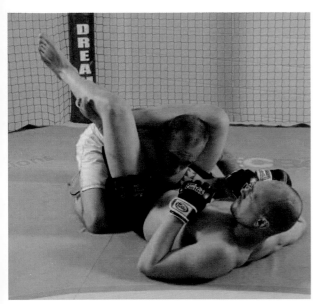

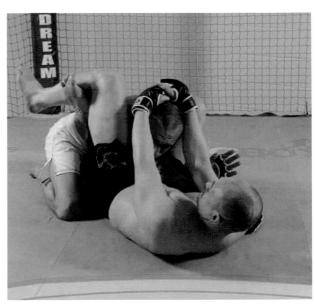

Fig 17.14 The fighter secures his leg around the opponent's neck, pulls the arm across and wraps the other knee around the other foot.

Fig 17.15 The fighter applies the triangle choke by pulling his knees together, raising his hips and pulling the head down.

INDEX